Healing Through Detox

Eliminating the Root Cause

of Chronic Disease

TAMARA ST. JOHN, M.B.A.

Healing Through Detox: Eliminating the Root Cause of Chronic Disease
Copyright @2017 by Tamara St. John
Published by Alternative Health Solutions Publications
P.O. Box 205, Rimforest, CA. 92378
ISBN 13: 978-0-9887671-4-0

Acknowledgments

I would like to thank God for helping me survive during my eight plus years of intense trial and illness and in the completion of this book. Thank you Lord for opening the doors of opportunity that no man can shut and for leading this book into the hands of millions so they can learn how to heal themselves.

I would also like to thank my parents for helping me during my long bout with chronic illness.

Praise for

Tamara St. John's Work

"Hi Tamara, just want to say thank you for all that you have accomplished and your book. You are a true pioneer in this field and it is very hard being a pioneer to open new ground and find new ways. Please do not stop what you are doing as it is helping so many people." **Craig Bowman, RHN, RNCP**

"I LOVE this book. I am a nurse & based on what I know & see I know that if I ever receive a cancer diagnosis I will NOT accept chemo & radiation to treat it. But as I've researched alternative medicine doctors I have learned that it can be very costly. Of course, you can research on your own & try to come up with a plan & "hope" that it will work. But that is a lot of work. This is a book written by someone who actually had cancer (a big difference, lots of books & info out there don't come from someone with firsthand knowledge & experience) & actually healed herself. And she is willing to share what she learned the hard way with the rest of us. This is truly a priceless book that I am so grateful to have in my personal library. And even though I don't have cancer, I also really love the detailed info on detoxing your body & I am following it currently. EVERYONE should have a copy of this book!" **Diane**

" Because of you & your book, I started on my journey back to natural health. I am now in remission of lupus & fibromyalgia. For just being the spring board in my life, I can't even begin to thank you enough!!!" **Vonda K.**

"Two months' cancer free now you and your book are a blessing from God" **Michael T.**

"I used many of the protocols in your book to help me heal serious ailments (not cancer) and it changed my life forever. I always refer back to your book when its detox time and it works wonders. 10 years of doctors and specialists couldn't do for me what your book did. My husband is even starting the detox regimen in order to get healthier. You are amazing and I thank you from the bottom of my heart." **Selena M.**

the second time this year. I'm feeling pretty good Tamara and shall be doing the kidney cleanse as from tomorrow. Last checkup found no lumps or increase in lymphocytes and the hematologist said; as I stand I have a normal life expectancy. I will be keeping on with the protocol till I am cured! Thank you so much...." **Jennifer H.**

"I have a testimony! Look I referred a friend to get your book that was diagnosed with Cancer 2 months. He called me and asked me for help. I referred him to purchase your book and to do all of the cleansers you suggested. Guess what his Brother just called me and told me he went back to the doctor and they said that the cancer was gone. They didn't see any signs of the cancer. He did everything in your book. Thank you so much you are healing people all over the world. Love peace and blessings to you!" **Drika B.**

"Your book is loaded with great information! I'm going to try the liquid Bentonite Clay and Psyllium Husk treatment for my first step in detox. I've known for years that I need to detox, but no one has had a reasonable plan and method for doing so. Thanks for writing this book!!!" **Judy I.**

"Thanks Tamara your book just saved my grandmothers life, she had breast cancer. We are from Jordan and I recommend everyone to use your book." **Samar J.**

"Amazing book I have read it twice and cured my IBS and hormonal imbalance from her knowledge in the book. A got to have book!" **Lori B.**

"Tamara, I just finished reading my copy - I loved this book - it is clear, concise, simple and straight forward - the plan you lay out anyone with even the smallest determination could easily execute. I am so thankful I found this book and you - and plan on reading (and re-reading) again and again. Thank you for sharing your journey and helping so many others!!! **Gia P.**

"I am amazed at the sheer amount of research that you had to do to bring this book to fruition and you are so generous in sharing. And to see that you included other testimonials in the book with other options is so selfless. You must be the angel that I have been praying for to enlighten me so I can help my friend. I am astounded at the depth of compassion you have to share what you had to research for yourself. I have to say again...thank you. When I lie down to go to sleep tonight, I will be thanking God that He led me to you." **Dianna M.**

"A must-read book, even if you don't have cancer. God bless you Tamara, you are an inspiration for others & you are serving and praising the Lord." **Joelle**

"Tam, I just received your book here in South Africa and its soooo awesome, I can't put it down...thank you, thank you, thank you, I'm immediately starting with some of your protocols and suggestions.... preventions are for SURE better than cure...love your book." **Debbie R.**

"I bought this book for my friend who is fighting cancer. It has given him fresh hope of beating this disease as full of so many ideas on how to use Gods natural medicine to heal the body. Another thing which has built his faith in Tamara's book is the fact that every consultant he has mentioned it to has endorsed it by saying he is doing exactly the right thing by following the advice given in her book." **Stephen Z.**

"I first heard Tamara St John interviewed a couple of times and was very impressed with her courage. I have been a follower on Facebook for a time now and couldn't wait to get her book. It is truly an inspiration to anyone whether or not they have cancer. I was certainly not disappointed with the book and I highly recommend it to all. A person needs this information so if a time comes when you have to make a decision for yourself or a person you care about, then you can make an informed decision." **Rachel H.**

"I have been following the author of this book on Facebook for two years, she's amazing! She has done more research on nutrition, the makeup of the cancer cell, and the root causes of disease than any medical professional I know. I have patiently waited for her to finish this book and read it within a few days of receiving it in the mail. I learned so much from it and it is definitely a resource I'll be able to utilize for a lifetime. I plan on buying this book for a few people I know who are suffering from various diseases, especially cancer. Highly recommend!" **Jessica**

Table of Contents

Author's Note

After I had published my first book; Defeat Cancer Now, on how I healed Cancer naturally and the steps I took to achieve better health through God's pharmacy. I was asked by many to write a book specific to detoxification and healing other diseases. This book is dedicated to those who suffer from many illnesses and want to know how to heal their body using detoxification and diet to gain freedom from chronic disease and achieve great health.

So why did it take me so long to follow up with my second book you wonder? Due to the extreme toxic environment and stress I was under during my bout with terminal cancer, my body had manifested other diseases which also needed to be healed naturally. This book will take you through my own journey of healing severe intestinal permeability, advanced adrenal fatigue, hormonal imbalance, small intestinal bacterial overgrowth (SIBO), auto brewery syndrome, food allergies and intolerances, asthma, and a comprehensive guide as to healing many diseases using proper detoxification methods and how to identify the root cause of your illness to find true health.

This book takes you through my personal journey to be better able to find your own root cause that is keeping you sick and how to heal the root cause so you too can achieve optimum health through God's Pharmacy.

1

Feeling Like "Job"

For those who have read my first book; Defeat Cancer Now, you are already caught up on the cancer battle which I experienced and the toxic overload which created other health challenges for my body. Throughout 2013; when my first book was published, I was still experiencing extreme food intolerances and allergic reactions, histamine intolerance, Irritable Bowel Syndrome (IBS), severe intestinal permeability (aka; leaky gut), low thyroid, extreme weight gain (80 lbs. in 8 months), estrogen dominance, auto brewery syndrome, asthma, small intestinal bacterial overgrowth (SIBO), adrenal insufficiency, and other issues. I had worked with Naturopathic doctors, doctors of chiropractic, and integrative doctors to see if I could get any help. All the while, I kept researching and experimenting on my own to try to heal my symptoms naturally.

By February of 2014, I was on my sixth doctor, a naturopath. I went to her and told her I had extreme leaky gut and severe food allergies and needed help to fix them. She had ordered a comprehensive stool analysis to diagnose the leaky gut, a very expensive $400.00-dollar test. I still had no insurance, so all doctor visits, supplements, and tests were coming out of pocket. When the results came back, the doctor told me that I had severe leaky gut. I told her; "tell me something I don't know, I already told you that in the beginning." I felt like I just wasted 400 dollars to tell me something I already knew. For anyone with severe leaky gut, the symptoms are obvious, with IBS and food intolerances or allergies. I spent thousands of dollars more for supplements that she recommended to heal the leaky gut, none of which ever worked for me. I told the doctor that her treatments weren't working and she got upset and fired me as a patient. This seems to happen more and more with doctors when they don't know how to help you, they blame the patient

1

and get rid of the patient instead of taking it as a learning experience to become a better doctor.

By September of 2014, I knew I was still very sick as I could now barely get out of bed and even the simple chore of taking a shower was a monumental task. My immune system had been suppressed with extreme inflammation and toxins for so long that my adrenal glands finally crashed. I ordered a full adrenal profile, which is a saliva test that gauges cortisol levels at four points throughout the day. I got the test back and brought it to an integrative doctor this time and she said that my adrenal fatigue was severe, which I already knew. The new doctor said she was impressed with all the research and work I had conducted into healing my body thus far but she didn't have anything further to add that could help me, so I left her office, after paying her hundreds of dollars for no advice, and decided that I was going to have to heal this on my own just like I had healed everything else.

By the end of 2014, I was exhausted and had a hard time functioning due to the adrenal fatigue. I had tried many different plans to heal adrenal fatigue and went to a couple more doctors to no avail. I finally decided to stop wasting my money on doctors who clearly didn't know how to heal anything. These doctors were practicing on me and I was paying them when I could practice on myself for free. I decided to save myself money, plus I didn't have all that much money to be throwing away on incompetent doctors.

I learned where to go to order the tests I needed and then heal myself naturally. I took the money I saved from going to doctors and spent it on an annual pass to Disneyland, figuring that Disneyland would be much better for my health than the incompetent doctors and dentists I had been going too, not to mention cheaper. I had tests done for my food allergies, tests for parasites, tests for adrenals, thyroid, tests for candida, tests for H. pylori, C. diff, cancer, etc., etc., etc. I had continued to heal my adrenal glands, severe leaky gut, biofilms, candida, parasites, and food allergies naturally.

When your adrenal glands are exhausted completely, it can take up to two years to heal. Within months of healing my adrenal fatigue, I was feeling much better with more energy. I also continued healing the leaky gut at this time as well since leaky gut and adrenal fatigue usually go hand in hand.

At this time, I felt it would be prudent to have all of my mercury fillings removed from my mouth because maybe that is what was keeping me sick. I sought out a holistic dentist who proceeded to remove seven amalgam mercury fillings in my mouth. Removing the mercury fillings didn't make much of a difference in my health, although my teeth did look better without all that metal. I also continued to detoxify my body for heavy metals during this time. I was diagnosed with periodontal disease many years ago, where the dentists I had gone too wanted to do root canals or remove my loose teeth and put in permanent ones. I had heard of how bad root canals would be for the body, so I opted to have nothing done and to try to heal the periodontal disease naturally. I was doing oil pulling (detoxification of the mouth) daily, healing biofilm infections, and keeping sugar to a minimum to keep my teeth intact.

By 2015, I had developed a severe tooth infection that wouldn't go away. I had continued to do research of periodontal disease, only to find out that periodontal disease is caused from a biofilm infection, which is impervious to antibiotics. The dentist gave me two separate types of antibiotics to get rid of the infection, but nothing worked. He told me that he wanted to remove my back teeth, but I was worried since I had recently lost a good friend to a massive heart attack a few hours after he had major dental surgery for advanced periodontal disease. I was fearful of the biofilm bacteria in the deep pockets of my teeth being moved around and hitting the bloodstream, thus causing major heart attack or stroke. I told the dentist that the antibiotics weren't working due to the biofilm which causes periodontal disease. The dentist got very upset with me and told me that "he was the expert and he had never heard of biofilms." So, I left that dentist since he didn't seem to be very knowledgeable about the scientific research already published in dental journals on the correlation between periodontal disease and biofilm formation. I decided to find out all I could and heal this infection myself, which took over 5 months to detoxify some of the biofilm formation causing the periodontal disease. Detoxifying from a biofilm from periodontal disease was the worst pain I had ever felt, which went from my left jaw all the way up to my ear with a throbbing, intense, stabbing pain all day long, every day for 5 months. I began to realize that the root cause of many of my health issues may be caused from the infections in my mouth and bone, so this was just another piece of the puzzle that I needed to heal.

In 2016, I had another tooth infection deep up into the bone due to the advanced periodontal disease and it could not be reached with the superficial biofilm and herbal treatments, so I had to resort to a different type of antibiotics which were injected into the gum line along the bone to try to kill the deep infection. At this point I began to realize that sometimes the infection can be so deep within the bone and that the infection is only one piece of the puzzle which was keeping me sick, regardless of eating a perfect organic diet and exercising.

I finally opted to go to another holistic dentist who referred me to an excellent periodontist, who was very knowledgeable regarding biofilms and periodontal disease. He had suggested laser treatment; to help remove the infection on the areas in my mouth plagued with advanced periodontal disease, to help to remove the infection and save most of my teeth. I finally ended up having to have the number 14 tooth removed and had laser treatment on all of my upper teeth to manage the infection. After the surgery, I had begun to feel much better, regaining more energy than I had in a long time. This was the first time in many years that my body began to respond to food again, where I could feel my body healing and responding to the organic foods I was eating, whereas before the laser surgery, my body didn't respond to anything I ate, no matter how healthy. The infection in my mouth was too great and what was keeping me sick.

Starting in 2016, I had started going back to traditional doctors to get tests done because I wasn't healing. My adrenal fatigue was getting better, but continuing to go to ignorant doctors and have needless procedures sent my adrenal glands crashing again by the middle of 2016, after I spent two years healing and was feeling tremendously better. I kept trying to tell these doctors about the infection in my gut (small intestinal bacterial overgrowth) and the periodontal infection which were both causing additional trauma and sickness in my body. These ignorant doctors refused to test me for infections in the gut because they said the testing for small intestinal bacterial overgrowth (SIBO) is not reliable, so don't bother testing. They also ignored my request to test for biofilm infections. These doctors didn't seem to want to do their job which did nothing to help me but only frustrated me further.

By January of 2016, my leaky gut was over 90% better, no more IBS, I could eat some of the foods I used to be allergic and intolerant too, and my adrenal glands were almost better as well. I was feeling great and healing until one day when I made a bowl of miso soup, and within ½ hour of eating this organic soup, my thyroid started itching and felt a bit swollen. I also had problems breathing and couldn't sleep all night long. I knew I was having an allergic reaction to the soy and that it further suppressed my thyroid function. I of course wasted my time by going to the emergency room where the doctors did nothing to help and seemed to have nary a clue what to do to make it better. So, I am back off all allergenic foods and I continue to monitor my diet making sure to only include foods that are healing and keeping any foods I used to be intolerant too, to a minimum. I am still healing for parasitic and biofilm infections within my body, continually detoxing out the root causes of my chronic conditions so they don't return.

This book will take you through my journey into the various stages of healing the body using alternative methods. This book will educate you on healing the body from within using diet, how to properly detoxify the body from the toxins that are keeping you sick, how to figure out the root cause of your illness and remove it, and how to heal yourself of chronic infections and disease.

In my quest to heal cancer and all of the other chronic health issues that I had experienced, I had become a better person and stepped into a career of helping thousands of others through my tragic circumstances. Although at times, I also believe that Satan was attacking me because he knows that God has a great plan for my life that would help millions of people. I know that God had put me into this situation of chronic illness to learn how to trust more in the Lord to direct me to learn how to heal everything naturally.

I believe that God gave everyone the ability to be able to "tune into" their body and to be able to listen to their body to heal naturally. My hope for anyone reading this book is that you stay positive through your fight and turn your trust toward the Lord. Rebuke Satan and your illness and thank God in advance for your complete healing daily. I am hoping that this book will help at least one person to survive their fight with chronic illness, learn to detoxify the body properly, heal naturally, and trust in the Lord for all your healing needs.

2

Why Are We Sick?

Ever since Richard Nixon declared the war on cancer in 1971, the cancer rates have skyrocketed to 1 in 3 women and 1 in 2 men who will get cancer in their lifetime. Aside from cancer, many more people have chronic illness and are taking daily prescription medications. People are popping their prescription medications per their doctor's advice, not realizing that those prescription meds will never heal their condition and the side effects can easily cause many other health problems.

America is the unhealthiest nation in the World and people continue to get sicker. So, what has happened in the last 45 plus years and why are we getting sicker than ever before? The answer lies in many different avenues; chemicals, sunscreens, radiation, genetically modified organisms (GMOs) in the food supply, pesticides, antibiotics, prescription drugs, illegal drugs, alcohol, air quality, and chemicals in the water supply, just to name a few.

Everywhere you turn, you are bombarded with chemicals on a daily basis. Most of you probably clean your home with chemically laced products, which you inhale on a daily basis. You use toxic chemicals daily in your shampoo, conditioner, lotions, skin creams, makeup, cologne, perfume, candles, room spray, toilet cleansers, bathroom & kitchen cleansers, supplements, vitamins, hair dyes, hair products, and sunscreen. I have been guilty of using some of these chemicals myself and some are difficult to avoid.

All of these toxic chemicals, you inhale into your body or put them directly on your skin, which is your largest organ. Everything you put onto your skin soaks into your bloodstream, which can cause health problems in the future. All of these chemical concoctions contain carcinogenic ingredients, meaning that they are known to cause cancer. Inhaling and putting toxic

7

chemicals onto your skin daily may eventually lead to toxic overload, which can cause many health problems. So how much sense does it make to slather on sunscreen, which contains carcinogenic ingredients, directly onto your skin? The sunscreen; which you have been told prevents skin cancer, is causing skin cancer. Some of you may even have mold or yeast growing in your home and are breathing in those toxins as well.

Another toxic substance to be aware of is the pollution caused by chemicals dumped into our air and water. Pesticides and herbicides are sprayed onto the food supply, which permeates the soil and eventually runs into the water supply, poisoning plants, animals, wildlife, and sea life. It is known that these pesticides and herbicides are toxic to the body and contain cancer causing chemicals. How long do you think you can ingest these chemicals without getting sick yourself? The labels on all of these pesticides state that they are harmful if swallowed and to call poison control if ingested. If you won't go drink pesticides straight from the bottle that they come in, why would you ingest it on your food or in your water?

Chemicals; such as fluoride, have also been added to the water supply. Fluoride is a known carcinogen that may cause cancers. Fluoride was also used in World War 2 to make the people docile, as it is easier to cull a docile population. Chlorine is also added to the water supply, in order to kill bacteria, but ingesting chlorine can't possibly be good for the body either. According to the Environmental Protection Agency (EPA); "Exposure to excessive consumption of fluoride over a lifetime may lead to increased likelihood of bone fractures in adults, and may result in effects on bone leading to pain and tenderness. Children aged 8 years and younger exposed to excessive amounts of fluoride have an increased chance of developing pits in the tooth enamel, along with a range of cosmetic effects to teeth." The EPA is admitting that excessive consumption of fluoride will lead to a variety of health problems. Of course, the EPA doesn't address all of the health problems associated with ingesting fluoride.

According to the EPA and reported by the Environmental Working Group; "there are over 316 known contaminants in our drinking water, with only 114 being regulated." Although, regulating the amount of chemicals that are safe for us to drink is ridiculous. No amount of toxic chemical is safe for us to drink. But we aren't just drinking it, we are inhaling it in the shower, bathing in it where it soaks into our bloodstream, washing our clothes in it, and washing our food in it.

Now that you are up to speed on the chemicals found in everyday products, chemicals in the water, and chemicals in the air, let's take a look at what has happened to the food supply in the past twenty plus years and how our food is making us sick.

Genetically Modified Organisms (GMOs), the brain child of Monsanto Corporation, are scientifically altered seeds to create a "bug resistant" superfood. Monsanto Corporation began tinkering with the food supply back in the mid-1990s; and since then, there has been an increase of people being diagnosed with allergies, asthma, cancer, diabetes, inflammation, autism, celiac disease, rheumatoid arthritis, and a host of other health conditions.

I am not saying that GMOs cause any of these health conditions, but the rise of health problems, which directly correlate with the introduction of GMOs into the food supply, cannot be ignored. Could GMOs be the reason for the rise in health issues? I know, from personal experience, that there is a definite correlation between the foods you eat and the state of your health. It has also been proven, by many people who change their diet, that eliminating GMOs from their diet, may correct many health conditions naturally.

I have personal experience with food allergies related to genetically modified ingredients. I have experienced allergic reactions to gluten, dairy, soy, corn and other genetically modified ingredients. After experiencing allergic reactions to many genetically modified ingredients, your body can even react to the organic version of those ingredients. I was even reacting to organic gluten, organic soy, and organic dairy. When I had cut out all genetically modified foods and their organic counterparts out of my diet, I began to slowly heal. Although, changing your food is only one piece of the puzzle to begin healing your body naturally.

Monsanto Corporation has been in the chemical business for many years and they were the company directly responsible for creating DDT; a pesticide used from the 1940s through the 1970s, until it was banned in the United States by the EPA. Monsanto is also responsible for creating Roundup Ready pesticide for crops, which is highly toxic. Monsanto is also responsible for Agent Orange; which is the chemical, known as Dioxin, which was sprayed on the residents and soldiers during the Vietnam War. Just in case you are not aware of the health problems, created by Agent Orange, inflicted upon the Vietnam veterans and citizens who were in contact with Agent Orange (Dioxin) during the Vietnam War, let me enlighten you. According to the Vets helping Vets website, "Symptoms of Agent Orange poisoning include; cancer, birth defects, chloracne, severe personality disorders, liver dysfunction, gastrointestinal disorders, kidney problems, neurological damage, psychiatric problems, metabolic disorders, cardiovascular issues, vision problems, and loss of hearing." Many of the offspring of those residents who inhaled agent orange, were born without limbs or organs due to the toxic effects of Agent Orange. Many of the Vietnam veterans had long term chronic health conditions

Monsanto is also responsible for creating Recombinant Bovine Growth Hormone (Rbgh) and Recombinant Bovine Steroid (Rbst), both of which are a type of hormone and steroid that is injected into cattle and chickens so they grow faster and can be slaughtered and send to market quicker than their organic counterparts. Due to the amount of people getting sick from the hormones and steroids that transferred into the milk supply, Rbgh and Rbst was banned for use in the milk supply and now most milk products come from cows not treated with Rbgh or Rbst. Although Rbgh and Rbst is still used in animals and transfers to the non-organic beef and chicken you consume. All of these chemicals are known carcinogens and may cause cancer and other health issues.

Apparently, poisoning the air, water, and soil was not enough for this monstrous chemical giant. Since the advent of the many toxic chemicals created by Monsanto Corporation, they have entered into the food business by altering the genomes of the seeds of the plant, known as Genetically Modified Organisms (GMOs). Here is an example of the way a genetically modified crop is altered to create a GMO. Let's take for example an ear of corn; the seed of the corn plant is spliced and mixed with fungicide, herbicide, pesticides, Agent Orange, bug parts, fungus, and mold and then put back together to grow a "super" corn that is able to withstand pests. Since the pesticide is injected directly into the plant itself, when a bug takes a bite of the food, their stomach explodes and they die.

The problem is that the bugs have become immune to these GMO crops and the chemical companies now need to create "stronger" GMO crops by increasing the pesticides they use within the seed of the food plant, hence the reason for adding Agent Orange to the new breed of GMO corn. If all of these toxic ingredients implanted into our food can make the stomachs explode in insects, which feed off of those plants, what do you think it is doing to you?

Since GMOs have been introduced in the 1990s, gastrointestinal disorders have skyrocketed, as well as a host of many other diseases. I am not directly blaming GMOs for the rise in gastrointestinal disorders or other disease, however I find the correlation of the introduction of GMOs and the rise of these gastrointestinal disorders to be interesting enough to write about. I personally cannot eat any GMOs, Rbst, Rbgh, or any other food that has pesticides or chemicals because I have extreme allergic reactions to them.   When you have gastrointestinal disorders, such as intestinal permeability, allergies and intolerances will increase exponentially.

Due to the toxic overload from detoxing too fast from a chronic condition, which created my intestinal permeability issues, when I have eaten any food with any GMOs, gluten, or dairy, I will have a histamine reaction show up on my face within 10 minutes of eating any chemically laden food. The allergic reaction was so bad that it formed a giant cyst near my nose and swells to affect my eyesight and my mouth. Sometimes the allergic reactions to food come in the form of large boils. Even after years of healing much of this issue, I still suffer from occasional food intolerances to gluten, dairy, soy and GMOs.

Currently the list of GMOs includes; Corn, sugar beets, cotton, zucchini, soy, Hawaiian papaya, alfalfa, and canola. GMO crops; such as, corn and soy, are made into various derivative ingredients that are put into processed foods. A few of the GMO ingredients that you will find hidden in the ingredient list of your favorite processed foods are; maltodextrin, soy lecithin, cottonseed oil, canola oil, whey, soy protein isolate, whey powders, high fructose corn syrup, corn syrup, corn sugar, aspartame, textured vegetable protein, soy sauce, tamari, NutraSweet, malt, soy milk, and many others. You will find a complete list of hidden GMO ingredients in a latter chapter. If you are interested in finding out more about GMOs in the food supply and how to avoid them, I suggest visiting the Institute for Responsible Technology website for the most up-to-date information. You can find that information at responsibletechnology.org.

If you currently have health issues and are interested in healing yourself naturally, start with what you are putting in your mouth. Cut out all GMOs, processed foods, non-organic meats, sugars, sodas, and other chemically laced food products. Just by changing the way you eat and what you put into your body will make a huge difference in the way you feel and begin to help your body to heal naturally.

Another major reason for chronic illness is from infections in the body that run rampant. Any infection in the body from gum disease, periodontal disease, H. pylori, small intestinal bacterial overgrowth, biofilms, candida, etc. can all cause further health issues. It is important to heal the infection first for proper detoxification to work effectively. If you find that detoxing the body or just changing your diet isn't working for you, check for infections and viruses within the body that may be keeping you sick.

After dealing with terminal cancer, the amount of toxins left over led to severe leaky gut, low thyroid, advanced 3C adrenal fatigue, small intestinal bacterial overgrowth, auto brewery syndrome, brain fog and more. I also experienced extreme weight gain where I gained 60 lbs. from juicing vegetables on a juice fast. For those with a chronic illness, it doesn't matter how healthy you eat, if your body isn't working correctly because you are NOT absorbing any nutrients! Most doctors (NDs, DCs and integrative included) aren't very helpful because they have NEVER been sick and are just practicing and guessing on how to heal you. Unfortunately, many health insurance plans won't cover natural therapies to heal your body and you are forced to resort to the traditional allopathic medical system, which is a real disservice to most of the population. It is best to tap into your natural born healing system; which is ingrained in all of us, and learn how to heal yourself if you ever expect to get well.

According to the American Journal of Homeopathic Medicine; "Antibiotics have long been known to suppress immune functioning." (1). This means that every time you take an antibiotic, it will not only kill the bad bacteria in your body, but will also kill the good bacteria which helps your body to function properly. Without the good bacteria in your body, your body will not be able to effectively fight off diseases or infections. If you take any type of antibiotic, it is imperative to replace your good bacteria with a good probiotic.

"With nearly half of all American adults have been diagnosed with at least one chronic health condition and this number is expected to increase in coming years." (1). This increase in chronic illness is in direct correlation with introduction of GMOs into the food supply, increased use/prescriptions of antibiotics, and increase in the vaccination schedule. One can only speculate that these factors are the catalyst to the declining health of the population. Think about this the next time you go to the supermarket to purchase your groceries, cleaning supplies, and other chemicals, start reading the labels and think about if you really want you and your family to be a human lab rat to the major chemical corporation.

3

Why Detoxification?

The first step to healing your body of any disease is to identify the root cause of the health crisis. Once you identify the root cause of what is keeping you sick, you can detoxify the body of those accumulated toxins; which can aid in eliminating the root cause which is keeping you sick. An accumulation of toxins lies in the colon, small intestines, digestive tract, blood, and tissue and may eventually lead to ill health and disease. Many times, the root cause of illness may be caused from candida overgrowth, biofilms, bacterial infections, viral infections, and/or parasitic infections. Once you get to the root cause of the problem and remove the toxins within the body, the body can begin to heal and repair itself.

Detoxification of the body will help to rid the body of the accumulated toxins that caused the illness or ailment in the first place. In order for detoxification to be the most effective, it should be done in a certain order to make sure the channels of elimination are clear to release the toxins. During detoxification, you may feel sick and lethargic, this is due to a Herxheimer reaction; also known as a healing crisis, which is discussed in detail in a latter chapter. Detoxification can make you feel as if you are coming down with the flu, but this will pass once the toxins are released from your body. During detoxification, it is imperative to get plenty of rest and drink plenty of water to flush the toxins out of your system.

How do you know if you are toxic? If you suffer from any of the conditions and symptoms listed in the box below, then you definitely need to detoxify your body. The proper order and various detoxification protocols will follow in later chapters. If you find you suffer from any of these symptoms of toxicity, you may also want to run some tests to pinpoint the root cause of your problems.

Symptoms of Toxicity:

- Fatigue
- Adrenal Imbalance
- Thyroid Imbalance
- Cold hands or feet
- Muscle Aches
- Lupus
- Joint Pain
- Chronic Fatigue Syndrome
- Neuropathy
- Epstein-Barr Virus
- Overall Bad Feeling
- Coughing
- Headaches
- Migraines
- Wheezing
- Poor Memory
- Mental Fog
- Depression
- Irritability/Anxiety
- Mood Swings
- Insomnia
- Hyperactivity
- ADD/ADHD
- Autism
- Vaginal Yeast
- Vaginal Itching
- Rectal Itching
- Menstrual Problems
- PMS Symptoms
- Endometriosis
- Infertility
- Hormone Imbalance
- No Sex Drive
- Cystitis
- Urinary Tract Infections
- Prostate Irritation
- Indigestion
- Protruding abdomen
- Eczema
- Psoriasis
- Athlete's Foot
- Cancer
- Swollen Lymph Nodes
- Colds and Flu
- High Blood Pressure
- Alzheimer's
- Dementia
- Parkinson's
- Blood or Mucous in Stool
- Autoimmune diseases
- Sinus Infections
- Post-Nasal Drip
- Ear Infections
- Itching
- Respiratory Problems
- Asthma
- Hay Fever
- Allergies
- Heartburn/Acid Reflux
- Gas/Bloating
- Diarrhea

- Constipation
- Ulcerative Colitis
- IBS
- Crohn's Disease
- Leaky Gut Syndrome
- Ulcers
- Intestinal Pain
- Chemical Sensitivity
- Dry Mouth
- Skin Rashes
- Hives
- Itching
- Boils
- Rosacea
- Dry Skin
- Bad Breath
- Burning/Puffy Eyes
- Dark circles
- Thrush (yeast in the mouth & throat)
- Fingernail/Toenail Fungus
- Over or Under Weight
-
- Low Blood Sugar (Hypoglycemia)
- Food Cravings (sugars & starches)
- Fibromyalgia
- Rheumatoid Arthritis
- Over sweating
- night sweats
- Diabetes
- Acne, Cystic Acne
- Fluid retention
- dark colored urine
- Inflammation
- Gingivitis
- Periodontal Disease

How to Detoxify the Body Properly:

There are many ways to detoxify the body and which method works for you will depend upon your level of toxicity and various health conditions. You see, one detox method may work well for one person but may not work well for another because everyone is trying to heal from different health conditions in which the root cause may be different and the levels of toxicity will vary from individual to individual.

One person may have infections, biofilms, and/or parasites which will cause chronically ill conditions in which it may take many years to detoxify the body properly, peeling away the layers of toxins and inflammation. Another person may only have mild toxicity and be able to detoxify the body in 30 days or less and see a huge difference. We are all different and no matter which case you are experiencing, you need to practice patience, which is much easier said than done. I myself have trouble with patience and have had to continually detoxify my body and stick to a very clean diet for over 8 years in order to completely heal my body of the chronically ill conditions which I had experienced and healed naturally through detox and diet.

I have had chronic infections, biofilms, candida, and parasites in healing leaky gut, advanced adrenal fatigue, and other chronic issues. It took me having to heal the gut lining first and getting rid of biofilm infections before my body began to respond to any of the detoxification protocols. The reason is that if you suffer from intestinal permeability (aka; leaky gut), detoxification will not work as well or sometimes at all because any supplement you take or food you eat is not being absorbed properly because it is escaping through the holes in the digestive tract and directly into the bloodstream. Also, if you have small intestinal bacterial overgrowth (SIBO), this can also hinder the detox process because your body is not working normally to detoxify properly. Even eating the healthiest foods can make your health worse because you cannot assimilate your food or the nutrients properly. Therefore, it can take years of healing the gut lining to be able to properly detoxify the body.

Once you have detoxified your body and begin to eat very clean and free from allergenic foods you may notice that you will be able to "feel" what is happening in your body. This is how you tap into the ability that God gave to everyone. God gave us all the ability to heal ourselves, but if you are constantly bombarding your body with toxic foods and chemicals, then your pathways are clogged. Once you unclog those detox pathways and start eating clean, you can begin to "feel" what happens in your body. Listen to your body, keep a journal if necessary, to identify what you eat while you are detoxing so you can begin to notice any patterns. Eating clean, detoxing the body and keeping a journal will help you to become more sensitive to what your body is telling you and you can tap into the God given ability to heal yourself.

So, if you have identified any of the symptoms of toxicity that you may have on the list, what can you do about it? There are tests that your doctor can order for you or you can order the tests yourself and conduct the testing at home to identify where your problem is so you know how to detoxify the root cause of the problem you are experiencing.

4

Testing Methods

I have been to over 20 doctors in the past few years and many of them weren't very helpful and a few of these "so-called" doctors even made me worse. I knew that I had to take my health into my own hands if I ever expected to get healed naturally from any of the conditions I was experiencing. One of the steps I took is to begin to test myself at home and then either take the results into a qualified doctor to read or to learn how to decipher the results myself and what they meant. Although I did end up taking some of my results into doctors, it mostly proved to be fruitless and I ended up having to learn to read the test results on my own.

If you find yourself going from doctor to doctor without success or find that doctors will not listen to you when you ask them to test you for certain conditions, maybe it is time you test yourself and bring the results into a qualified doctor for interpretation or learn how to read the test results yourself. It really isn't difficult to learn how to read the results yourself and you may surprise yourself with your new-found knowledge.

Here are a few of the tests which have been helpful to me over the years. These are also tests that do not need a doctor to perform so you will be sent the test kits in the mail and can do the test at home and then send them into the lab. These are the same exact labs that doctors can utilize when ordering test kits for you, you are simply omitting the middleman.

The Navarro Urine Test:

John Beard, PhD and embryologist had proven in 1902 that the trophoblast cells present in early pregnancy are nearly identical to cancer cells. Both emit the hormone called human chorionic gonadotropin, also known as HCG. HCG is the substance that protects the fetus from the mother's immune system and also protects the cancer cells. According to G. Edward Griffin, author of "World without Cancer", "The greater the malignancy, the more these tumors begin to resemble each other, and the more clearly they begin to take on the classic characteristics of pregnancy trophoblast."

In 1974, Dr. Virginia Livingston and her researchers also discovered the same HCG hormone existing in both pregnant women and those with cancer. According to William Fischer, "Sadly, Livingston's discovery of the growth hormone wasn't taken seriously until scientists at Rockefeller University, Princeton Laboratory, and Allegheny General Hospital in Pittsburgh isolated it in lab samples."

In the late 1950's, Dr. Manuel D. Navarro, an oncologist, had developed a test which would detect the presence of cancer within the body. The Navarro urine test is based upon the scientific theory that the trophoblast cells in pregnancy and malignant cells both display the human chorionic gonadotropin (HCG) marker. This means that cancer patients showed the same HCG markers as that of pregnant women. This test has been proven to be 95% effective in detecting cancer. The 5% of people who had inaccurate test results were of those who had "false positives" and all later had gotten cancer. Therefore, the test seems to be much more effective than 95%.

Although many people use this test to determine if their cancer treatments are working, it can also be used to detect cancer up to two years in advance. According to the Navarro Medical Clinic website, "The test detects the presence of brain cancer as early as early as 29 months before symptoms appear; 27 months for fibro sarcoma of the abdomen; 24 months for skin cancer; 12 months for cancer of the bones (metastasis from the breast extirpated 2 years earlier)." So this would be a great method for early detection so one can change their diet, detoxify their body and possibly avoid a future cancer diagnosis.

Dr. Efren Navarro, the son of the late Dr. Manuel D. Navarro, now runs the clinic in the Philippines and continues his father's work. When testing for the presence of HCG, to detect cancer, you must make sure that you aren't pregnant first. For women, you must abstain from sexual contact for 12 days prior to performing the test and for men; you only need to abstain from sexual contact for 48 hours before performing the test. If you are currently taking thyroid medication, hormone pills, steroid compounds, a smoker, or vitamin D, it is advised to stop taking these for 3 days prior to performing the urine test so it doesn't affect the results. The urine test is done at home and is very affordable and easy to do.

To perform this test, you will need:

- An unbleached coffee filter (brown)
- A glass jar
- A glass measuring cup with the cup, milliliter, and ounce measurements
- Pure Acetone (nail polish remover will NOT work); get this in the paint department at your local hardware or specialty store.
- Rubbing Alcohol
- Measuring spoon
- Plastic sandwich bag

You may have most of these items already in your home; however, if you do not, you can purchase them for around $10.00 U.S. at your local Wal-Mart, paint store or hardware store. Make sure to look in the paint department for the pure acetone, as nail polish remover will not work.

On the day of the test, take 1.7 ounces (50 ml) of first morning urine and add 7 ounces (200 ml) of acetone and 1 teaspoon (5 ml) of alcohol into a jar and mix well. Close the jar and put into the refrigerator for at least 6 hours, until you notice sediments have formed on the bottom of the jar. After 6 hours, pour off half of the urine mixture, without disturbing the sediment at the bottom, and re-close the jar. Shake up the sediment mixture and pour into a coffee filter to capture the sediment within the urine. Let the coffee filter air dry, indoors, until the sediment is dry. You would then fold up the coffee filter and put into a plastic bag before sending the sample to a lab in the Philippines, where it is tested for the presence and level of HCG.

The scale in which to measure the levels of cancer within the body are easy to read. A level of 1-49 I.U. is considered negative for the presence of HCG and 50 I.U. and above is considered a positive reading for HCG. This test will be able to tell the level of cancer within the body although it should be correlated with other test results. I highly recommend visiting the Navarro medical center website, which can be found at www.navarromedicalclinic.com to find out more information about the Navarro urine test, the cost, and address of where to send your sample.

Even though I knew that I had cancer due to the extreme symptoms and the presence of the Epidermal Growth Factor Receptor rash, I still had people doubting that I ever had cancer at all because I wasn't diagnosed through the traditional method. I guess I can't blame them for being so conditioned into believing that if you don't look sick, or you haven't lost your hair from toxic chemotherapy treatments, or a traditional medical doctor hasn't diagnosed the condition, then it must not be true. That is exactly how western medicine and the pharmaceutical companies have conditioned everyone to believe. The point is, when you have advanced cancer, you definitely know it is there, there is no denying the advanced symptoms.

I wish I would have known about this test in the beginning of my cancer in 2009, but I didn't. So, after having enough of the negative comments from people, who doubted my having cancer to begin with, I decided to take the test to see if I still had cancer. I still felt the presence of cancer within my body due to lethargic symptoms that closely matched the symptoms I had previously, so I conducted the urine test in March of 2012, where I used my first morning urine to test. After a few weeks, I received my results via email and this was the actual email I received from the lab:

Dear Tamara,

Your HCG Test Result on 03/31/2012 is:

Index + 4, (52.6 Int. Units)

This is within the POSITIVE range (0 I.U. - negative, 1 to 49 I.U. - doubtful [essentially negative], 50 I.U. & above - positive). A POSITIVE result indicates the presence of Human Chorionic Gonadotropin, a hormone found in the urine of pregnant women. Numerous medical reports show this to be present in the urine of cancer patients. However, the result must be correlated with the medical information (X-rays, CT Scans, Ultrasounds, MRIs, etc.). A biopsy procedure confirms the diagnosis of cancer. The elevated HCG is possibly coming from remnants (microscopic or otherwise) of the breast cancer. This serves as the baseline result.

Results can go up to 10,000 int. units or more especially in testicular cancer, some uterine cancers (H mole and choriocarcinoma) and germ cell tumor. However, most other cancers have results anywhere from 50 to 80 or 90 IU. The result must be correlated with the medical history together with other pertinent medical information (X-rays, CT Scans, Ultrasounds, MRIs, etc.). The test cannot determine the stage of the cancer but when it is done on a serial basis, say once a month, one can follow and monitor the progress of the disease.

Wishing you the best of health, I remain.

Sincerely Yours,

Efren F. Navarro, MD

My Test Results:

According to my test results, it shows a 52.6 reading with a +4 marker. This indicates a definite positive reading for HCG (Human Chorionic Gonadotropin). Since I was definitely not pregnant, it means that I still had remnants of cancer within my body. Since my symptoms were much worse physically, with visual symptoms, in 2009 and 2010, this reading shows that my cancer is decreasing and what I have been doing thus far has been healing cancer naturally. Since I now had a positive result for the presence of cancer, I now had proof to those people who refuse to think outside of the box and realize that when cancer is in the advanced stages, there is no denying it because the symptoms are clear. I knew of a woman who was diagnosed with terminal cancer by traditional methods and she also took the Navarro urine test to track her progress. Her number was below mine, sadly she died a few years ago. Below are pictures of how to do the Navarro urine test, these are my personal samples from when I conducted the test in March of 2012.

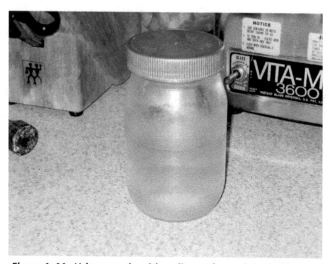

Figure 1: My Urine sample with sediment formed on the bottom

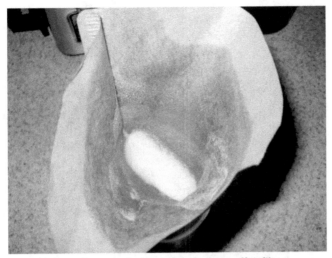

Figure 2: poured mixture into brown coffee filter

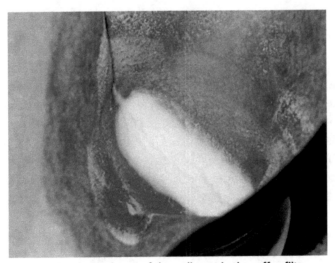

Figure 3: Closer picture of the sediment in the coffee filter

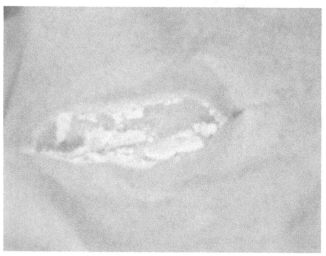
Figure 4: dried sediment after it sat out for a few hours.

Comprehensive Stool Analysis:

There are different forms of the stool analysis. The comprehensive stool analysis tests for fungus, candida, parasites, digestive function, H. pylori, C. diff, bacterial counts, and markers for inflammation. The comprehensive stool analysis can be added with parasitology for one, two, or three days consecutively. The kit is sent to you to take samples from your stool daily and put it into vials, which is then sent to the lab for analysis. These tests are very expensive, but worthwhile, and can tell you A lot about your health. I had gotten this test done from www.labtestsplus.com.

I have found that the parasitology portion of the test is not very accurate, so it is best to do the three-day testing to hopefully catch any parasitic activity you may be experiencing. Although, parasites are very elusive and even the three-day stool test can be negative for parasites even though you may still have parasites, so do not take the stool test results as the end all, be all, of testing. I have also found that some of the parasites seen today have suctions (ropeworms) that will attach themselves to the intestinal lining and not let go while they are alive, which is another reason that parasites are so elusive and will not always show up in a stool test. These parasites have to be killed before they expel themselves into the stool, more on how to get rid of parasites in a later chapter. Parasites also seem to be more active around the full moon and/or new moon, so it may be better to schedule this test with the full moon cycle so you have a slightly better chance of the parasites showing up in the stool sample.

After you receive your stool test kit in the mail, here are a few tips to make it easier for you for collection of the stool sample for testing. Make sure to have some heavy-duty gloves on hand, heavy duty paper plates, plastic forks & knives to be able to do this test properly without too much trouble. I find it is easiest to put on the plastic gloves and put the paper plate over the toilet bowl and then release your stool onto the paper plate. The reason for the heavy-duty paper plate is that the test will come with a small paper flimsy thing that you are supposed to aim perfectly and hope to not make a mess. The heavy-duty paper plate will make it much easier to collect your sample without making a mess. Once you receive your results, you will be able to take it to a qualified doctor to read them or they are pretty easy to read yourself.

Functional Adrenal Stress Profile:

If you find you are extremely fatigued, or maybe you have anxiety symptoms, or panic attacks, you should take the adrenal stress profile to find out if your adrenal glands are over taxed. This test is sent to you with four empty vials and a set of directions. You are to spit into each vial at certain times of the day. This will tell you what your cortisol levels are at each time of the day.

This test cost around 300 dollars, but in my opinion was very worth the money as it told me a lot about why I was feeling so horrible. Also, it tells you where on the scale you fall in terms of your adrenal function. You cannot heal adrenal fatigue successfully without first knowing whether or not you have high cortisol levels, normal cortisol levels, low cortisol levels, or completely crashed. Knowing where you stand can help to put you on the road to recovery. This test can also measure DHEA levels, Estradiol, Estriol, Progesterone, Testosterone, and Melatonin.

Testing Saliva for cortisol is much more effective than the Cortisol blood test given by a traditional doctor. The blood test for cortisol will only measure whether or not you have Cushing's disease or Addison's disease; these are the two opposite ends of the Cortisol spectrum. The blood test will not tell you the many stages in between the two, which may cause many health problems. When your adrenal hormones are imbalanced, the other hormones follow suit and will also become imbalanced. The Saliva cortisol test is a great tool to have to bring the results into your qualified naturopathic or functional medicine doctor to assess how to heal your body naturally.

Intestinal Permeability (Leaky Gut):

There are multiple ways to test for intestinal permeability. Comprehensive stool analysis can test to see how well the food is digested and the levels of good to bad bacteria in the digestive tract. There is also a urine test to test for leaky gut; although not recommended for diabetics, which will test for how well the small intestines are absorbing food.

I personally like the comprehensive stool analysis because you can see how much good bacteria you have in your stool. When I took the test in 2014, my lactobacillus (good bacteria count) levels were not measurable, meaning I had none. I also had very low levels of bifido bacteria (another good guy). It was also found that I had higher levels of biofilm bacteria in my digestive tract. This test was invaluable in
helping to diagnose extreme intestinal permeability (leaky gut) and target another piece of the root cause of my health problems.

Small Intestinal Bacterial Overgrowth (SIBO):

There are breath tests which also test for the presence of small intestinal bacterial overgrowth (SIBO). When you test for SIBO, the test should measure both hydrogen and methane levels. Many breath tests for SIBO only measure hydrogen levels and if you are one who is a methane producer, you can get a false negative because the methane gobbles up the hydrogen causing a negative result, when really you may be positive for methane producing SIBO. So, before you order a SIBO testing kit, make sure that it does test for both hydrogen and methane so you can get an accurate reading.

Some gastroenterologists also will test for SIBO, but I have unfortunately found a lack of knowledge regarding SIBO in the traditional gastroenterologist. You can find the SIBO test kit at commonwealth labs or quintron labs. I am sure there are other companies who offer the SIBO breath test, check your prices, that the test measures BOTH hydrogen and methane, and which labs they are sent too.

Commonwealth labs has a SIBO test which tests both hydrogen and methane, which you can order yourself and send in to be tested. However, the best test for SIBO is the lactulose breath test and this specific test does need to be ordered by a doctor. I had to end up testing myself for SIBO because every time I asked a doctor to test me for SIBO, they would make up excuses why they couldn't test. After getting the run around from multiple lazy doctors who didn't want to do their job, I finally found a lab where I could test myself and skip the lazy, unknowledgeable doctors.

Food Allergies and Intolerances:

Many people have multiple food intolerances or allergies, so it is important to test for intolerances and/or allergies to pinpoint exactly which foods may be causing the health problems. There is the celiac antibody panel, the Food IgG, and urinary peptides tests which will detect for food allergies and intolerances.

The Celiac antibody panel is a dried blood spot assessment which evaluates for IgG and IgA to wheat gluten (gliadin); which can isolate Gluten Sensitivity, but also Total IgA and Tissue Transglutaminase (tTG) antibody as well which is more specific for celiac. The Food IgG is a finger prick blood test that tests for over 90 different adverse food reactions.

The Urinary Peptides test evaluates for the presence of elevated peptides (brain toxic chemicals) to gluten (found in wheat and wheat related products) and casein (found in cow dairy). Peptides from these food sources are known to trigger behavioral and language difficulties in individuals with an autism-spectrum disorder. (labtestsplus.com)

I had personally taken the IgG test for food intolerances and what I found most difficult about this test is that you have to fill up rather large circles on a lab testing card with your blood. So, it is a finger prick test but I had to invite my friend over to do the finger pricking for me, because I get faint and hyperventilate at the sight of needles. Needless to say, I was hyperventilating and crying and she ended up having to prick my fingers about 30 times just to get enough blood to fill up the circles on the lab testing card.   I was mentally exhausted afterward and administering this test was quite an ordeal, although the test results were very informative.

My personal test results showed my intolerance to gluten, dairy, soy and also a measurable amount of brewer's yeast candida in my blood stream (auto brewery syndrome) which had caused multiple occasions of becoming legally drunk from eating a plate of brown rice and vegetables.

Tissue Mineral Analysis:

This test is very helpful in measuring your mineral levels and ratios. The worst part of this test is that you have to cut a piece of your hair next to the scalp to be sent into the lab and tested for the levels of 29 different minerals and 8 different heavy metals. This test is helpful for anyone suffering from chronic illness, chronic fatigue, thyroid issues, adrenal insufficiency, heavy metal exposure, hair loss, memory loss, headaches, insomnia, and copper toxicity or if you are having problems healing naturally and want to find out which minerals you are lacking. You can order this test directly from UniKey health, information in the appendix section.

The most helpful part of this test is that the results are accompanied by 20 pages of lifestyle, supplement and dietary recommendations related to your specific results interpreted from Ann Louise Gittleman. This test was very helpful to me in finding out which mineral imbalances I needed to focus upon in order to begin healing properly.

MTHFR Mutation:

MTHFR is an abbreviation for Methylenetetrahydrofolate Reductase. I will be using the abbreviation for obvious reasons. The MTHFR gene is a genetic mutation in which your detox pathways will not be working normally so some people may have a more difficult time ridding the body of toxins. A genetic test can be done at home via saliva is through www.23andme.com where you send in your saliva sample and they give you a lot of raw data all about your genetics. Once you have gotten your results back, you can upload those results to http://geneticgenie.org to help you read the results. So, if you find that detoxing isn't helping you, you may want to try this test to see if you have a MTHFR defect.

These are just a few of the tests which you can do on your own without seeing a doctor first. I am not telling you to skip a doctor altogether and take matters into your own hands, however that is what I had to end up doing with my own health if I ever wanted to get better as doctors were not helping me and many were making me worse with their supplements and bad dietary advice.

I also find more and more people without the funds to be able to afford healthcare, lack of funds to see a qualified doctor, or on the highly-flawed welfare healthcare system; which contains some of the worst doctors in the world. Many times, it is imperative to learn to listen to your body and heal yourself, which may be the only way you can heal properly instead of relying on ignorant physicians.

5

Barriers to Detoxification

This chapter is specifically for the many people out there who are chronically ill and are not improving regardless of the healthy foods they eat or the fact that they keep trying to detoxify their bodies. There are various ailments in which detoxification or ingesting healthy foods will not improve your health. The following is a list of some of these ailments:

Intestinal Permeability (Leaky Gut):

For those who have read my first book and have been following me, you know that terminal cancer had caused many other health issues for me. One of them was severe leaky gut which I have been dealing with for over 5 years now. I knew I had leaky gut back when I had cancer, but I was officially diagnosed with severe leaky gut in February of 2014. I have been healing leaky gut naturally for years and I can attest that it is no easy task and takes a lot of time and patience. I have researched, experimented on myself, read many books, journal articles, and attended long-winded summits; most of which were written by well-meaning doctors or researchers who have never had leaky gut. Of course, those of us with leaky gut that follow their advice become very frustrated at their lack of knowledge regarding leaky gut and how to heal it naturally.

In order to detoxify your body properly so you can begin to heal your body naturally, you need to heal the lining of your gut first. If your gut is already in good shape and you are not allergic to any foods and are absorbing the vitamins and minerals from the foods you eat, then you can skip to the detoxification chapters and begin with the detoxes.

When you have intestinal permeability (aka; Leaky Gut), the food you eat doesn't fully digest, and whole food particles will permeate through the holes in the small intestines and leak into the blood stream, which may cause food allergies, food intolerances, auto-immune diseases, boils, rashes, Rosacea, Eczema, and many other health conditions. In the beginning stages of intestinal permeability, it is difficult to notice any symptoms, aside from a few allergic intolerances to food which may go unnoticed.

As your intestines become more permeable; the holes in your intestines become larger and it may lead to, autoimmune diseases, extreme allergic reactions, Crohn's disease, hives, attention deficit hyperactivity disorder (ADHD or ADD), inflammatory bowel disease, irritable bowel syndrome, rheumatoid arthritis, chronic fatigue, migraines, lupus, fibromyalgia, autism, ulcerative colitis, eczema, psoriasis, rosacea, skin problems, schizophrenia, Alzheimer's, Dementia, small intestinal bacterial overgrowth (SIBO), and celiac disease. Your stomach may also protrude, making you look pregnant when you aren't. This is due to the bad bacteria in your gut, which overtakes the good bacteria.

Intestinal permeability can be caused from antibiotic use, systemic candida, parasites, vaccines, overabundance of toxins, chemotherapy, radiation, alcohol, and drug use. Due to some people having intestinal permeability, it is important to heal the gut lining if you expect to be able to absorb any nutrients from your food or supplements. You also may not be able to eat many foods due to extreme food allergies or food intolerances.

Symptoms of Intestinal Permeability (leaky gut):

- Food Intolerance (Gluten, Dairy, Soy, Corn, Chocolate, Eggs, Nuts, etc.)
- Food Allergies (same list as intolerances)
- Celiac Disease
- Histamine Reactions (swelling, edema, inflammation, asthma)
- Irritable Bowel Syndrome (IBS) or Irritable Bowel Disease (IBD)

- Ulcerative Colitis
- Crohn's Disease
- Adrenal Fatigue
- Autism
- Diarrhea or Constipation
- Small Intestinal Bacterial Overgrowth (SIBO) or Gas/bloating
- Abdominal Pain
- Memory Loss
- Mood Disorders (Anxiety, Depression)
- Fatigue
- Rashes
- Eczema, Rosacea and skin infections
- Auto Immune diseases
- Alzheimer's/Dementia

If you are showing any of these symptoms, it is possible that you may have leaky gut. Leaky gut can be caused from Candida overgrowth, Parasites, eating Genetically Modified Foods, Vaccine Damage, overuse of antibiotics which kills all good bacteria leaving an imbalance, NSAIDS, anti-inflammatory medication, etc. Any of these things can disturb the balance of good to bad bacteria within the gut and lead to dysbiosis and overgrowth of candida and/or parasites. Candida and parasites can end up boring holes into the small intestinal walls and then you are no longer able to absorb nutrients from the food you eat, no matter how good of a diet you have.

It was very easy to tell when I had leaky gut as my symptoms were severe, although I have since healed it naturally and many of my food allergy symptoms. The minute I would eat any offending food; such as gluten or dairy, I would be running to the bathroom less than a minute later with Irritable Bowel syndrome (IBS). Within 10 minutes of eating an offending food, half of my face would experience facial edema and blow up like a balloon where the swelling would close my eye and lip on one side of my face. The food allergies, histamine reactions, and IBS were extreme and it was very obvious that I had leaky gut.

I finally had the money a few years later to go to the doctor and get a test done. I told the doctor that I had severe leaky gut and she suggested that I spend 400 dollars on a test to confirm my diagnosis. The doctor came back after seeing my test results and told me that I had severe leaky gut. I told the doctor; "tell me something I don't know..."

What I can tell you about leaky gut and healing is that you absolutely need to stay away from ALL offending foods and you cannot cheat at all or it will set your healing back. Get a food intolerance test (IgG test) done to find out what your food triggers may be. You will not be able to heal leaky gut if you continue to eat those offending foods.

After a few years of avoiding all of the offending foods, I did re-introduce a couple of the foods I was previously intolerant too. I was able to eat a bit of sprouted bread and some dairy, as long as it was from raw goat's milk or raw sheep's milk since those are easily digestible. When I tried to re-introduce soy, in the form of homemade miso soup from organic soy, my thyroid began to itch within a half an hour and I started having breathing problems, extreme cold feeling, and throbbing aching all over my body in my joints. I realized that I still have major problems with soy as it is goitrogenic and I was diagnosed with low thyroid years ago. Eating the soy further suppressed my thyroid for the moment, but in a few days, I warmed back up and the thyroid stopped itching. So, I remain staying away from ALL offending foods.

Secondly, taking supplements in pill form are a complete waste of your money because if you have severe leaky gut; you will not be able to absorb the pills anyways because the outer coating is too difficult for your gut to digest in its permeable state. Any supplement you take must be in powdered or liquid form only. You can open some supplement capsules to get the powder out of them. Make sure that when your doctor suggests supplements for leaky gut, they need to be in powdered or liquid form only or make sure that you only purchase capsules that can be opened and emptied out.

If you have leaky gut, you may have a problem with some of the detoxes in this book until your leaky gut has healed. This is why I added the chapter on leaky gut because you have to heal the gut lining first for the detoxes too work effectively. What I found most frustrating while trying to heal leaky gut is the sheer amount of misinformation out there from doctors and researchers who have never had leaky gut. I had tried all their suggestions to no avail, so I finally came up with a plan that worked for me to heal severe leaky gut and get rid of most of my food intolerances and histamine reactions. I am still very careful in what I eat and still do not eat gluten, dairy, or GMOs but I do cheat on occasion, none of us are perfect. Meaning, I can eat a bit of organic gluten in the form of sprouted grain bread and won't experience any histamine reaction, Rosacea, IBS, brain fog, etc. where before I used to experience all of those symptoms even with organic gluten.

I have literally been to over 20 doctors, all of which were less informed on how to heal my body. I even had one doctor who actually said something brilliant; "she said that I needed to find a doctor who was smarter than I was." She was right AND I still haven't found one! What I can tell you is that the majority of the doctors and their books are a waste of money and most doctors (allopathic, functional, and naturopathic) are clueless as to how to heal leaky gut. A few of these doctors even made my condition worse by their suggestions and supplements.

What I can tell you is this: leaky gut is very tricky to heal because everyone has different issues which may have contributed to the leaky gut. Some of us may also have infections; such as, C. difficile (C. diff), H. pylori, small intestinal bacterial overgrowth (SIBO), parasites, candida, and all have a type of yeast overgrowth within the digestive tract which may or may not be candida (there are many strains of candida and yeast that can cause health issues).

Also, if you have periodontal disease or infections in the mouth, it is very common to have infections in the gut as well. You need to get rid of the infections in your body to completely heal the body because severe infections will overwork your immune system and keep the body sick. Because all of our bodies are different and we each have different health issues to deal with; you need to listen to your body and YOU know your body better than any doctor ever will!

Here is the plan that I created to heal leaky gut which has worked for me. With severe leaky gut, you cannot absorb ANY type of pills as they just pass through the holes in your digestive tract and into your bloodstream, so you will never reap the benefits and you are wasting your money on expensive supplements. STOP wasting your money on the expensive pills sold by doctors who have no clue! Give your body the building blocks to heal in the form of bone broths, powders and liquids only!

Healing Leaky Gut, Ulcerative Colitis, Irritable Bowel Syndrome (IBS), and Crohn's:

Step One: If you are dealing with severe leaky gut; like mine was, you need to start healing the IBS, IBD symptoms first: I used turmeric spice in the powdered form ONLY; NO PILLS!!!! I took 1 tsp of turmeric powder in a few ounces of water up to 3 times per day. This got rid of the severe IBS symptoms within weeks. You add 1 tsp of turmeric to a few ounces of room temperature water and stir briskly until mixed. Drink quickly like a shot and follow up with some water to wash down the taste. If you find that you are getting a headache with 3 tsp of turmeric per day, scale back the dosage. The headache you may feel is a sign that your liver is overburdened with toxins, so drink plenty of water to flush the toxins.

Some researchers say that you need to add black pepper or oil to turmeric for it to be absorbed into the body more effectively. You DO NOT need to add black pepper or oil, as turmeric works perfect on its own, God did not need to add black pepper but made turmeric work great all by itself. I have tried it both ways and have found absolutely no difference in effectiveness by adding black pepper. However, if you "feel" that the black pepper makes the concoction more absorbable then by all means add some black pepper.

The Turmeric increases glutathione production within the body and glutathione is the master detoxifier of the body. I explain glutathione in more detail in the chapter on Liver Cleansing. I also bought my turmeric in bulk since buying the spice on the spice isle in the grocery store becomes too expensive. I find bulk turmeric at Middle Eastern grocery stores is much less expensive than any traditional grocery store.

Step Two: Bone Broth daily. I used to drink bone broth at least 3 times per day for breakfast, lunch, and dinner. I could not absorb or eat anything else at the time as I couldn't digest or absorb anything. Your body will tell you what it needs to heal, listen! If you have issues with bone broth due to the histamine levels, you may do better with homemade chicken broth where you just cook the whole chicken or parts of the chicken down to the bone.

If you can absorb or eat vegetables, then by all means do so, but raw vegetables may be too harsh on your system, so steam your vegetables lightly and chew the vegetables well until they are almost mush. I know that I personally couldn't digest raw vegetables well at all, so I had to leave them out. I even had to refrain from cooked vegetables for quite a while because my body wouldn't tolerate them, so just pay attention to what your body is telling you.

After more than a year of healing the gut, I am now able to eat well cooked vegetables in my soups. I always have a crock pot of soup available for a quick meal during the week.

Bone Broth Recipe

- Soup bones or beef marrow bones

- 3 tsp of Bragg's Apple Cider Vinegar

- Himalayan Pink Salt to taste

- Water

In a crock pot, put the soup/marrow bones, apple cider vinegar, and pink salt. Fill the crock pot with water and turn the crock pot on low. You can also use a regular pot on the stove. Whether you use a crock pot or regular pot, this process takes approximately 12 - 24 hours of cooking time, sometimes I do more and you will notice the bones breaking down and the marrow has released from the bone and into the broth. Once finished, put the broth into refrigerator and sometimes the mixture will become gelatinous; which is what you want to happen. This is very healing and a great base broth for vegetable soups if you can digest cooked vegetables.

If you have problems with the bone broth due to histamine levels, you can use a whole organic chicken or organic chicken parts in its place. I will often use a few chicken legs or turkey legs.

Step Three: L-Glutamine in powdered form only. You do NOT need to buy the expensive powders sold online from doctors. I buy my L-Glutamine powder from vitacost (ARO brand) and use 5 -10 grams, 3 times per day, mixed in smoothies or juices. If you only have the L-glutamine in capsule form, then open up the capsules and add them to your smoothies.

I have created a meal replacement smoothie which includes L-Glutamine for those who cannot digest whole foods or just to make your life easier to combine all of the ingredients at once. See the recipe at the end of this section.

Step Four: Aloe Vera Juice. ONLY use the liquid form from George's Always Aloe Vera or Lily of the Desert brand. I have tried both, but like the Lily of the Desert brand best, as it has helped me to heal the most. I use the "stomach" formula and the "detox" formula of the Lily of the Desert brand. The detox formula can help to detoxify your body while also healing the gut lining because it isn't as harsh on the digestive tract due to being in liquid form.

Step Five: Licorice Root powder. This will help to heal the gut lining. You can get pure licorice root powder from mountain rose herbs. Be careful on dosage as this will raise blood pressure naturally. Once your body can handle pills, you can switch to DGL or licorice pills; I take 1 DGL pill, 3 times per day before meals. DO NOT take licorice if you have high blood pressure, are on blood pressure medication, or are pregnant or nursing.

The benefits of Licorice are many; "including **asthma, athlete's foot, baldness, body odor, bursitis, canker sores, chronic fatigue, depression, colds and flu, coughs, dandruff, emphysema, gingivitis, tooth decay, gout, heartburn, HIV, viral infections, fungal infections, ulcers, liver problems, Lyme** disease, menopause, psoriasis, shingles, sore throat, tendinitis, tuberculosis, ulcers, yeast infections, prostate enlargement and arthritis." (3).

Licorice contains glycyrrhizin; which can cause high blood pressure, salt and water retention, and low potassium levels, which could lead to heart problems. DGL products are thought to cause fewer side effects because the DGL is a form of licorice with the glycyrrhizin removed so therefore may be safer. (2).

The DGL comes in a tablet form and needs to be chewed until it is liquid and the licorice is supposed to aid in healing the lining of the digestive tract. I never noticed a big difference from using the DGL tablets, but did it anyway before each meal.

I have created a meal replacement smoothie which includes licorice for those who cannot digest whole foods or just to make your life easier to combine all of the ingredients at once. See the recipe at the end of this section.

Step Six: Slippery Elm Bark. "The mucilage comes from the inner bark of the tree and is a bit slippery and slimy, hence the name "Slippery Elm". The mucilage does a good job of soothing and coating the mouth, throat, stomach, and intestines, causing much relief from things like Gastroesophageal Reflux Disease (GERD), Crohn's Disease, ulcerative colitis, diarrhea, diverticulitis, and Irritable Bowel Syndrome (IBS)." (4).

Slippery elm will not be absorbed well unless in powdered form. Slippery elm is an added ingredient in the lily of the desert aloe vera juice. You can also get powdered form of slippery elm from mountain rose herbs or vitacost. Once your leaky gut improves, you can begin to take the slippery elm in pill form, but I still find it easier just to add it to my morning smoothie so I take less pills. I add 1 tsp of slippery elm powder to a morning smoothie daily. This ingredient will make your smoothie a bit thicker, so don't let that smoothie sit around or it will be too thick to drink.

I have created a meal replacement smoothie which includes slippery elm for those who cannot digest whole foods or just to make your life easier to combine all of the ingredients at once. See the recipe at the end of this section.

Step Seven: Probiotic enemas. Only use powdered probiotics and do a probiotic enema. This will help right away with IBS, IBD, Crohn's, and ulcerative colitis to get the good bacteria back into your colon. I use Natren's brand of powdered probiotics, they carry a non-dairy formula for those who are sensitive to dairy.

Probiotic enemas are meant to be retention enemas, meaning you hold the liquid in your colon and keep it there for as long as possible. So, get something to read and relax in the bathroom while you are lying down on your side giving yourself the retention enema. I found this helped tremendously with the IBS symptoms by increasing the good bacteria back into the colon.

Probiotic Enema

This enema will help to restore functionality to the colon, heal the intestinal lining, and restore good bacteria within the colon and lower intestines.

Mix together:

- 1 tsp Natren's Digesta Lac Powder
- 1 tsp Natren's Bifidofactor Powder
- 1 tsp Natren's Megadopholous Powder
- 1 cup Lily of the Desert or George's Aloe Vera Juice Stomach formula
- ½ cup of Cold Pressed Flax seed Oil

Once mixed in a bowl, mix with a wire whisk and pour into a clean enema bag. Make sure to perform a cleansing water enema or coffee enema prior to using the retention enema to clear the colon of fecal matter. Put a bit of coconut oil on your rectum or on the tip of the enema tube or both, whichever you find the most comfortable. Lay on your right side and insert the tip of the enema tip into your rectum, open the spout of the enema tube and let the retention enema flow into your colon. The point is to retain the enema contents as long as possible until it soaks into the colon. Try to hold it in at least a couple of hours, but if you can't, you will still be getting some healing from it.

I have also performed a retention enema with only the probiotic powders and water; start with a small amount and work your way up. If you start with too much probiotics in your colon, you can experience a massive "die-off" reaction that will give you intestinal cramping, bloating, gas, and/or burping for hours. Start with small dosages and work your way up to the larger dosage.

You should also be taking probiotics internally so you are getting the intestinal benefits from both ends and re-populating your gut with good bacteria and healing the colon at the same time. However, if you have a severe leaky gut condition, make sure the probiotics are in powdered form as pills will not be effective because they will pass through the holes in the gut. Natren's or VSL #3 are the only companies I know of that carries an excellent brand of powdered probiotics that are either with or without dairy, although these probiotics can be pricey.

After healing any severe leaky gut condition, you can switch from powdered form of probiotics to pill form probiotics and your body will tell you when you can handle that stage. I prefer Prescript Assist probiotics in pill form.

Step Eight: Probiotics orally. You may have to wait on this until your body can handle it. Again, if you are severe, DO NOT take probiotics in pill form as they will NOT work. I have wasted thousands of dollars on probiotics in the pill form that never did anything to improve my situation. Powdered probiotics are the only form that can help leaky gut. Natren's and VSL #3 are the best brands I have found that are in powdered form. Only switch to pill form once your gut has mostly healed and you can absorb the pill form and then you must switch up the probiotic strains and formulas, so don't stick with one brand.

If you only have probiotic capsules, open them up and empty the powder from the capsules into a smoothie. I still open up the capsules and put them into a smoothie because they are easier to take then swallowing a bunch of pills. Also, don't start with a large dosage of probiotics as it is a waste of money. When your body is depleted of probiotics and you are trying to re-build the good bacteria in your body, start small. Open a capsule and only take ¼- ½ of the probiotic powder, saving the rest for another day. Introduce the probiotics into your body slowly, to be able to handle an increase in good bacteria, without overwhelming your system.

Some people swear by getting your probiotics from food; as in sauerkraut or yogurt. However, sauerkraut is a high histamine food and many people with leaky gut cannot handle foods with histamine, I know I certainly couldn't. If you find you can handle sauerkraut, then it is best to get your probiotics from food such as raw sauerkraut daily or the sauerkraut juice. It took me a long time of healing the gut before I could digest or handle the histamines from sauerkraut. So, this is individual as to what will work for you, either probiotic powders, sauerkraut, or a combination of both.

The brands of sauerkraut that are the best are Bubbies at www.bubbies.com and Saverne. You can find Saverne at www.krautlook.com and it has different flavors of their raw sauerkraut. I personally hate the taste of traditional sauerkraut, but I find the flavors of the Saverne sauerkraut more interesting and palatable for my taste buds. Make sure to chew the sauerkraut completely until it is mush before swallowing to get your digestive juices flowing and get the full effects of the probiotic power.

Yogurt is also tricky for many with leaky gut due to dairy intolerances. I personally couldn't handle dairy for many years due to the dairy intolerance. If you don't have an issue with dairy, make sure your yogurt is organic from both grass-fed cows and cows not treated with Rbst/Rbgh. However, now you can find almond and coconut milk yogurt on the shelves, as well as kefir, Kombucha, and lassi at various markets.

Step Nine: When you can handle solid foods, make sure to cook all of your vegetables well or put them in a soup broth until soft. Chew all of your food until it is mush to trigger the digestive enzymes within your body.

Digestive Enzymes are imperative before each meal, but when you have severe leaky gut, you may not be able to handle digestive enzymes. Again, you will need to open up the capsules and put the powder into a smoothie until your digestive tract can process the pill form.

My favorite digestive enzymes are the Doctor's Best brand of Digestive Enzymes. The reason I like this brand best is due to the high protease count that it contains. When you have a high protease count in a digestive enzyme, it helps to digest proteins, including parasites (which are made up of protein) which may be plaguing your system. Also, these digestive enzymes don't make my stomach burn as other digestive enzymes often will. It all depends upon your specific needs.

If you cannot handle solid foods, I have created a smoothie recipe at the end of this section to aid in healing your gut.

Step Ten: Another key to healing the gut and detoxifying the body properly is making sure to lessen the effects of histamine reactions within the body. Histamine is supposed to be carted out by the body, but sometimes there are certain factors which cause histamine to build up within the body causing swelling and allergic (histamine) reactions. I have had major problems with histamine reactions over the years due to severe leaky gut and SIBO conditions, but with continued detoxification, healing my gut lining and diet changes, the histamine reactions are kept to a minimum when I stick to the diet religiously.

Keep to these ten steps and you will experience relief from Irritable bowel syndrome and Intestinal permeability and your body will begin to respond to detoxing methods again. Another essential tip is too support the liver while you are healing, add liver healing foods (see Liver detox chapter) to your diet or smoothie to help you heal quicker.

Be Patient!!! This is easier said than done. You need to realize that severe leaky gut will take YEARS to heal properly and it is very frustrating. You have to stick to a non-GMO, no processed foods, no sugar, no offending foods (gluten, dairy, eggs, etc.) and you cannot cheat or it will only prolong the healing process. Once you heal, keep to a healthy, organic, non-GMO, non-processed, and no sugar diet. Eventually, you will be able to re-introduce some offending foods in time, but you still want to be very cautious because if you do have a reaction to a specific food, it can set you back on your path to wellness.

I have created a smoothie to help with healing leaky gut and this can be used as a meal replacement for those who are having problems digesting whole foods. You can use this smoothie in addition to the bone broth and 10 steps above.

Leaky Gut Smoothie

- 1 scoop Now Foods **Pea Protein** Powder (I prefer the Dutch chocolate but you can also use the unsweetened formula or a different flavor.)

- 2 scoops (1 tsp-1 TBS) of ARO brand **L-glutamine** powder (vitacost)

- 1 scoop (1 tsp) of **slippery elm** powder (mountain rose herbs)

- 1/8 tsp of **spirulina powder** (mountain rose herbs) or 1 tsp of **KyoGreen** powder (if not allergic to gluten or barley).

- 1 tsp of **licorice root** powder (leave this out if you have high blood pressure or advanced adrenal fatigue)

- 1/8 tsp of **maca root** powder (only use a little bit unless you have severe adrenal fatigue and then skip it until your adrenals heal a bit more)

- Unsweetened Silk Vanilla **Almond Milk or Water**

This smoothie is also good for a meal replacement for those who are having problems digesting or absorbing any type of food. Once your gut heals enough, you can start to go into the detoxes to purge the candida and parasites that are most likely the root cause of the leaky gut.

Histamine Intolerance (HIT):

Some of the reasons that your body creates too much histamine are due to high estrogen levels or estrogen dominance, because estrogen stimulates histamine. (5).

Another reason for histamine intolerance is the body is not producing Diamine Oxidase (DAO) within the intestines and the DAO is what suppresses excess histamine from entering the body. Intestinal Dysbiosis, Small Intestinal Bacterial Overgrowth (SIBO) or leaky gut are factors which may also cause high histamine levels and histamine reactions.

Eating high histamine foods; such as sauerkraut, cured meats, and red wine, will also increase histamine levels and can cause histamine reactions in someone who is already histamine intolerant. Histamine is naturally supposed to clear out of your system but some reasons that histamine may not be clearing out is due to estrogen dominance, a deficiency in progesterone, using birth control pills, deficiency in vitamin B6, Small intestinal bacterial overgrowth (SIBO), lack of DAO, and/or a genetic mutation, such as the MTHFR defect.

The way to detoxify your body of the histamine levels is too avoid the high histamine foods; such as, aged cheeses (bleu cheese, etc), cured meats, cured fish, bone broth, fish stock, chocolate, red wine, champagne, vinegar, and all fermented foods. This was very difficult for me as many of these items were my favorite foods and drinks that I would crave daily. It is also imperative to avoid any foods that may cause sensitivities, which are mainly gluten, soy, dairy, corn, wheat, eggs, and nuts.

It is also necessary to improve gut functionality as having leaky gut will hinder proper detoxification of the body. Not only does having leaky gut hinder detoxification, but it also hinders histamine from leaving your body. This is why I had heavy histamine reactions where my face would blow up like a balloon only 10 minutes after eating an offending food that I was allergic too. Not only was I diagnosed with estrogen dominance and low progesterone but also with severe leaky gut.

Supplementing B-6 can help, although if you have severe leaky gut, no supplement in pill form will help and it is best to get the supplementation from liquid or powdered form as well as food. Vitamin B-6; also known as pyridoxine, is important for the breakdown of fats, proteins, and carbohydrates. (6)

Foods high in B-6:

Liver	Green Beans	Bananas
Wild Fish	Chicken Breast	Turkey
Grass Fed Beef	Carrots	Eggs
Walnuts	Sunflower Seeds	Avocado
Dried Beans	Hazelnuts	Garlic
Cooked Spinach	Whole Grains	

Some of the few foods I could tolerate at the height of my severe intestinal permeability ordeal were not only the chicken, turkey, or bone broth but I could also manage to eat avocados safely. If you have problems tolerating some of the foods high in B-6 on this list, you can always soak the nuts and seeds and then blend them into a smoothie.

One test you can do to find out if you are histamine intolerant is a food allergy test. If your food allergy test comes back positive, you may not have histamine intolerance and your issue may be food allergies. However, if you are having intolerance to specific food items and your food allergy test comes back negative, that is a sure sign of a histamine intolerance issue.

This had happened to me where I used to have a positive food allergy test and had worked my way through the years of healing that. However, I was still experiencing food intolerances to gluten, dairy, and soy. I did get another food allergy test in 2016 which came back negative, indicating that I did in fact have histamine intolerance. According to the allergist who was treating me, there is currently no testing for histamine intolerance.

To help reduce the histamine reactions, I began taking a Histamine Blocker by Nutricology called DAO Histamine Digester or Seeking Health also has one called Histamine Block. I have discovered that if you take at least 10,000 HDU of diamine oxidase (ingredients in some histamine blockers), 15 minutes prior to eating high histamine foods, you will not have a histamine reaction or the histamine reaction will be lessened greatly. The pills are pretty pricey, which is why I stay on a low histamine diet and only take 1 pill when I want to eat something that may cause a food reaction.

Another reason for food intolerance histamine reactions can also be due to small intestinal bacterial overgrowth (SIBO). There is a new supplement on the market called Atrantil, which was invented by a gastroenterologist. I have found that Atrantil can help with lessening bacterial counts in the small intestines and helps to lessen the effects of histamine reactions. Although the one drawback is it is a bit pricey for those who need to take it full strength (6 pills per day) to rid your small intestines of bad bacteria. I took it for 1 month and found it did help a little, but I would need to take it much longer to make a difference and it wasn't that affordable.

Another supplement that helps to reduce the histamine in the body is Quercetin/Bromelain, in addition to digestive enzymes prior to eating. I find that the Quercetin/Bromelain works just as well as the histamine blocker capsules and is much less expensive. I take 1,000 mg of Quercetin/Bromelain three times per day before meals.

Adrenal Fatigue:

Another barrier to detoxing the body properly is adrenal fatigue and many don't realize that if you have adrenal fatigue, you will most likely have leaky gut, thyroid imbalance (hypo/hyper) and other hormonal issues as these go hand and hand. Adrenal fatigue or Adrenal insufficiency is not yet recognized by western medicine due to their insufficient testing methods and general ignorance by traditional doctors.

Cortisol is the stress hormone; released by the adrenal glands, which regulates the changes that occur in the body; such as, (3)

- Blood sugar (glucose) levels
- Fat, protein and carbohydrate metabolism to maintain blood glucose (gluconeogenesis)
- Immune responses
- Anti-inflammatory actions
- Blood pressure
- Heart and blood vessel tone and contraction
- Central nervous system activation

Cortisol levels are supposed to fluctuate throughout the day with the higher level being in the morning and this is the reason why you are able to get out of bed with energy in the morning. The lowest level of cortisol fluctuation is in the evening, which is why it makes it easier to fall asleep.

However, when the stress hormone cortisol is over-working itself due to long term illness and/or stress, then the adrenal glands can become fatigued. You will generally find that you may have high cortisol levels for a length of time before your adrenals become fatigued to the point of having consistently low cortisol levels throughout the day. When your cortisol levels remain high for too long, the cortisol levels will eventually exhaust themselves.

Currently, western medicine guidelines only test cortisol levels using a blood test and do not recognize anything aside from Cushing's and/or Addison's disease as being an adrenal problem. According to WebMD; Cushing's syndrome is when your cortisol levels are too high and Addison's disease is when your cortisol levels have flat lined and your adrenal glands have failed.

There are levels in between Cushing's and Addison's which are very serious and need attention because it is those levels in between which are the road directly to Cushing's or Addison's. You don't just wake up one day with Addison's, there will be years prior in which your immune system is severely compromised and cortisol levels may start out high but then eventually crash and end up on the lower end of the spectrum veering toward Addison's disease.

When your immune system is compromised for any length of time, you are at risk for adrenal fatigue and possible adrenal failure. I was personally diagnosed with severe adrenal fatigue back in October of 2014 where even getting out of bed or taking a shower became a monumental chore as I was running on empty without any energy whatsoever. A simple shower would make me feel like I worked a 10-hour shift.

It is not safe to detoxify your body during an adrenal crisis and you must first heal your gut and immune system enough to be able to withstand the rigors of a detox. For years, since I was diagnosed with severe leaky gut and adrenal fatigue, my detox pathways seemed to be blocked and I couldn't detox properly until my gut lining was healed and my adrenals were almost healed. Here are my test results for adrenal fatigue diagnosis taken back in September 2014:

Functional Adrenal Stress Profile Plus V – 205

Parameter	Result	Reference Range (units)
Cortisol - Morning (6 - 8 AM)	6.0*	13.0 - 24.0 nM/L
Cortisol - Noon (12 - 1 PM)	3.0*	5.0-8.0 nM/L
Cortisol - Afternoon (4 - 5 PM)	2.4*	4.0 - 7.0 nM/L
Cortisol - Nighttime (10 PM - 12 AM)	1.1	1.0 -3.0 nM/L
Cortisol Sum	12.5*	23.0 - 42.0 nM/L
DHEA-S Average	11.11*	2.0 - 10.0 ng/mL
Cortisol/DHEA-S Ratio	1.1*	5.0 - 6.0 Ratio

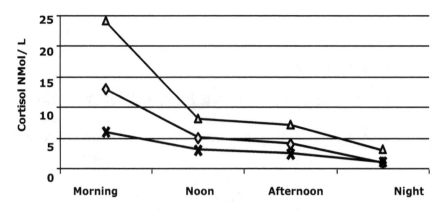

Figure 5: Triangle = High Cortisol level, Diamond = Low Cortisol level, X = My Cortisol Level. September 2014.

As you can see from my test results, the top line with the triangle indicates High Cortisol levels, the middle line with the diamonds indicates Low Cortisol levels and the bottom line with the x's were my cortisol levels; back in September of 2014, which are below the low level. My total cortisol sum was at a 12.5 back in September of 2014. Once you get to this point, it isn't much further before being diagnosed as full Addison's disease which may lead to sudden death.

I had re-taken the test in February of 2015 and my total cortisol sum was at a 39; with my morning cortisol being 31 of that number (highly elevated), but much improvement from the previous sum of 12.5. The total sum of Normal cortisol salivary levels should be between 23 and 42 (depending upon the lab, this number could vary slightly).

I had been healing adrenal fatigue and leaky gut naturally for a few years before I was able to detoxify my body properly. With adrenal fatigue, I focused upon getting more salt into my system through a salty concoction called Sol'e (pronounced Soul-aye). Sol'e is when you fill a mason jar about 1/3 full of pink Himalayan Salt or Celtic Salt and then fill the rest of the jar with pure filtered water and shake until the two are incorporated. Let the mixture sit on your counter for 24 hours, shaking occasionally, and you will notice the salt will dissolve a bit into the water. Then use 1-2 TBS of this salt mixture (called Sol'e) into a regular glass of water and drink this mixture whenever you drink water until you begin to feel better. I was drinking Sol'e for the first 5 months and really craving salt, so don't be shy and sprinkle the salt on your food as well. After 5 months, the Sol'e didn't taste good to me any longer and I was beginning to feel much better. Again, this is an instance where you need to listen to your body and what it is telling you. Also, whenever my adrenals felt exhausted again, I would re-start the Sol'e water until I felt better.

I had read every single book on adrenal fatigue and can tell you that none of their suggestions worked for my situation. Many of the books were not addressing the root cause and were ignoring the fact that most everyone who has adrenal fatigue usually also has an intestinal permeability issue and possible SIBO infection.

Eating more carbs; in the form of sweet potatoes or potatoes, did help to give me my energy back. Normally, I wouldn't eat that many carbs but when you have adrenal fatigue, specific dietary restrictions may go out the window in order to feel better. I still needed to steer clear of gluten, sugar, dairy, caffeine, alcohol, processed foods and GMOs. If you have severe adrenal fatigue; as I did, it can take up to two years to heal completely and every single case of adrenal fatigue that I have studied all had the leaky gut component with it. So, while you are healing adrenal fatigue, you also need to be healing the leaky gut.

Adaptogenic herbs can be helpful for some people with mild adrenal fatigue, but for others with severe adrenal fatigue, the use of adaptogenic herbs can make you crash harder and make your condition worse. Adaptogenic herbs are those herbs that help the body to normalize physiological functions amid stressful conditions. Many of these herbs can lower or raise cortisol levels, but use them cautiously. The adaptogenic herbs consist of ashwagandha, holy basil, maca, licorice root, astragalus, rhodiola, ginseng, chaga mushroom, cordyceps mushroom, to name a few. Many of these can lower cortisol naturally and produce a calming effect and may be beneficial if you are in the beginning stages of adrenal fatigue with high cortisol levels. However, if you have advanced adrenal fatigue, where your cortisol levels are very low or crashed, even a small amount of an Adaptogenic herb can make you wired and then eventually make you crash harder. Be very cautious when using these herbs and know the level of your adrenal fatigue before taking any adaptogen. There are also many doctors out there touting their adrenal formulas, which contain adaptogens, which may or may not be beneficial for your specific condition. I had many doctors who suggested I take their "adrenal supplements" but they always made me feel much worse due to the adaptogens used in their supplement formulas and my advanced adrenal condition.

If you have adrenal fatigue, you also want to look for the root cause of the reason that your adrenal glands are being overworked. For many it is stressful situations, like a death in the family, finances, work pressures, or a prolonged illness. For me, the catalyst was prolonged illness and infections in the body that were overworking my immune system and adrenal glands to cause them to eventually crash. Chronic illness puts undue stress upon your body, so it is imperative to learn to de-stress yourself when trying to heal your body naturally.

Healing Adrenal Fatigue:

1. **Find the root cause** of your adrenal fatigue and work on healing the root cause. (Prolonged illness, infections, stress, leaky gut, etc.). If you have adrenal fatigue, you also may have a leaky gut issue, work on healing both. The leaky gut smoothie recipe works well for adrenal fatigue.

2. Add **Sol'e** to your diet; drink the salty water all day long until it no longer tastes good to you.

3. Add **healthy carbs** back into your diet. If you are diagnosed with adrenal fatigue, going low carb can be your worst enemy. Put those carbs back into your diet. Potatoes really helped me to heal. I added more sweet potatoes and regular potatoes to my diet. Also, lots of cooked vegetables.

4. **DO NOT** go overboard with adaptogenic herbs. The adaptogenic herbs can cause your body to crash harder if you

have a severe adrenal fatigue, borderline Addison's disease. If you are in stage 1 or 2 Adrenal
Fatigue, you can probably handle a few adaptogens. Stage 3 and 4 Adrenal Fatigue should never be taking adaptogens as it can make your condition worse.

5. Do the **Adrenal Healing Smoothie** daily as this will replace the vitamins and minerals in your body helping you to get stronger quicker. (See recipe below).

Adrenal Healing Smoothie

- 1 scoop Now Foods **Pea Protein** Powder (I prefer the Dutch chocolate but you can also use the unsweetened formula.)

- 2 scoops (1 tsp-1 TBS) of ARO brand **L-glutamine** powder (vitacost)

- 1 scoop (1 tsp) of **slippery elm** powder (mountain rose herbs)

- 1/8 tsp of **spirulina powder** (mountain rose herbs) or 1 tsp of **KyoGreen** powder (omit KyoGreen if you also have SIBO due to the prebiotic content or are allergic/intolerant to barley/gluten).

- 1 tsp of **licorice root** powder (leave this out if you have high blood pressure or have advanced adrenal fatigue)

- 1/8 tsp of **maca root** powder (only use a little bit unless you have severe adrenal fatigue and then skip it until your adrenals heal a bit more)

- Unsweetened Vanilla **Almond Milk** (Silk brand is my favorite) or **Water** to make a drinkable shake

- ½ tsp of Himalayan fine pink **salt** or Celtic sea salt (fine).

It was the combination of this daily smoothie, the Sol'e and adding back in the carbs which helped me to regain my energy and strength and get rid of adrenal fatigue. I still need to be cautious of my stress levels and not too overwork my body (difficult for my type A personality) so as to keep a balance.

Small Intestinal Bacterial Overgrowth (SIBO):

Small intestinal bacterial overgrowth; commonly called SIBO, is a condition in which the small intestines harbors a bacterial infection. The bacteria that should normally be in the large intestines have made its way into the small intestines and have become overgrown. The bacterial infection in the small intestines causes many health issues; such as, extreme bloating (looking pregnant), rosacea, eczema, rashes, absorption problems, vitamin and mineral deficiencies.

I had this condition during the time I had leaky gut. You will find that if you have SIBO, leaky gut usually accompanies this as well. Because your gut function isn't working well, it allows for bad bacteria to get trapped in the small intestines causing further health problems. This health challenge was the hardest thing I have ever tried to heal from and was much more difficult than healing terminal cancer.

It doesn't matter what you are eating if you have SIBO, you can have the healthiest diet in the world and it will not make a difference as the bad bacteria in your small intestines feeds off every food group, no matter how healthy. SIBO will also feed off probiotics, prebiotics, Kombucha, and all fermented foods. There are people who think that if you just eat healthy and get plenty of probiotics that it will starve the bad bacteria, they are sadly misinformed.

I went for many years of people telling me that my problem was my diet, when nothing could be further from the truth. I had been to countless doctors, gastroenterologists, allergists, pulmonologists, cardiologists, etc. When I asked the gastroenterologist and other doctors to test me for SIBO, they told me that the test wasn't effective so it wasn't worth testing for it. I was shocked, none of these doctors wanted to help me or do their job. Refer to the testing chapter for information on testing for SIBO.

Healing Small Intestinal Bacterial Overgrowth (SIBO):

1. **Support your liver:** drink lemon water daily and add liver detoxing foods and supplements to your diet. This is a must as you will be eradicating the bacterial overgrowth from the intestines and the liver detox pathways need to be clear to help facilitate the amount of toxins which will pass through the liver.

2. **Take herbal antibiotics daily**: Berberine, Allicin (Allimax Pro), Neem, Oregano Oil, Olive Leaf Extract, Peppermint Oil (Peppogest), Atrantil.

3. **Support Motility**: MotilPro (Pure Encapsulations), Iberogast.

4. **Fasting Diets:** These are extreme measures, but if you can handle the taste, this will help to heal your SIBO within 21 days and may need to be repeated to make sure the SIBO is gone.
   - Vivonex by Nestle (not suggested due to the high cost and horrible genetically modified ingredients).
   - Homemade Elemental Diet (less expensive, better ingredients, but tastes horrible).

5. **Low Residue Diet (FODMAP):** If you choose to continue to eat and forego the fasting diets in point #4, make sure to eat a low residue (low FODMAP) diet consisting of foods that are less likely to feed the bacterial infection. You will find the FODMAP diet in a later chapter. Although my SIBO problem was so severe that not even eating low FODMAP helped my condition, so this is dependent upon the severity of your condition.

6. **Keep a positive mindset:** See yourself well and you will begin to heal. You will find more information on the mind/body connection in a latter chapter.

For me, healing SIBO was a catch 22 scenario. Doing Low FODMAP ended up cutting out many carbs, which made my adrenal fatigue worse when I went too low carb. If everything I ate was feeding this beast inside of me, then I just decided to stop eating and conduct water fast (I do not suggest this method). I ended up doing multiple water fasts throughout 2013 to help rid my body of the SIBO and heal leaky gut. However, due to my weakened immune system from the cancer; water fasting ended up causing severe adrenal fatigue, although it got rid of much of the SIBO. I do not suggest water fasting for those with compromised immune systems and many people with SIBO will have a compromised immune system because your gut is harboring too much bad bacteria and therefore not functioning properly.

When I conducted multiple water fasts throughout 2013, I noticed that I had an extreme amount of burping. So much so, that I ended up keeping a journal tracking the number of burps I had daily while on the water fast. In the beginning of the water fast, I was burping over 100 times per day and it got less each day as the bad bacteria left my body. I ended the water fast on day 33 with about 14 burps per day. I also lost over 30 lbs. and my pregnant looking belly really decreased. Fasting was not easy and I was thinking about food constantly. My favorite hobby became drooling over all of the menus online for all of my favorite restaurants.

I did try the homemade elemental diet later and do agree that it is the best method, but the taste is so awful that it is really hard to get past it. You are still fasting, but your body is being supported with the elemental diet due to the amino acids, dextrose and salt. You are keeping up your bodily functions but not feeding the bacterial overgrowth.

A safer method to get rid of SIBO is to continue to eat the low residue (low FODMAP) foods, take herbal antibiotics, deal with motility issues, support the liver and keep a positive mindset.

Underlying Infections:

Another barrier to healing the body can be found in other infections in the body. There are fungal infections, viral infections, bacterial infections, parasitic infections and biofilm infections. If you find that your detoxification efforts are not working for you, you may want to look deeper into any infections that may be hindering your progress.

I had found that the root cause of many of my health problems from cancer to leaky gut to SIBO and more were all caused from the advanced periodontal infections eating away at the bone and spreading to other parts of my body. I also had the infections in my small intestines (SIBO) which I took care of, but I was still experiencing health problems. I still had an asthma like condition where I could no longer walk a flight of stairs, a hill, or walk too fast without becoming out of breath with my chest hurting. It wasn't until I addressed these specific infections where my body began to heal and I was able to detoxify my body again.

Fungal, Parasitic and biofilm infections will be addressed in upcoming chapters. You can have tests done from your doctor to verify if you have a viral, parasitic, fungal or bacterial infection that may be keeping you sick. Although many traditional doctors may not be convinced or they are not educated enough to be looking for the root cause of any disease because they only treat the symptom. It is best to find an integrative doctor or naturopathic doctor to help you find out if you are harboring any of these infections that may be keeping you sick.

After you have healed leaky gut, adrenal fatigue and any infections within the body, then you can start the detoxes to get rid of the other root causes of disease. Some other root causes which may be causing your health issues are infections, candida, biofilms and parasites, which are discussed in detail in the following chapters.

6

The Colon Cleanse

The Colon; also known as the large intestines, contains muscles where the stool is formed and pushed along the walls of the colon. Billions of healthy bacteria line the walls of the colon keeping it in perfect balance. However, due to ingestion of toxic food and antibiotics killing good bacteria, the bacteria in the colon can get out of balance and cause disease and death, which can begin in the colon. Over time, not eating the proper food can lead to constipation issues where toxic material from the feces is trapped in the colon. The longer the toxic waste stays in your colon, the greater chance of developing disease. This is why it is important to detoxify your colon on a regular basis. A healthy person will experience bowel movements at least 2-3 times per day with ease. If you are not experiencing ease of bowel movements at least twice per day, then you may be holding toxic waste in your colon that can create sickness and disease in the future. It is imperative to rid your colon of that waste in order to return your body to a healthy function. The reason to begin with the colon cleanse is that you want to clear the channels of elimination that are keeping you sick. Once you clear the colon, the other cleanses will go easier because you have cleared the colon of toxic debris first.

When beginning a colon cleanse, there are many different types to choose from. You can either use liquid Bentonite clay and Psyllium Husk taken daily and every evening or you may use a kit that is usually found in any vitamin or health food store. All of the colon cleanse kits will work differently because everyone's body chemistry is different, so it is difficult to say that one kit is better than another. The kits usually work when you take a combination of pills per day according to the instructions on the box.

I will sometimes opt for the detox kit, but I also utilize the liquid Bentonite Clay/Psyllium Husk method. With the Liquid Bentonite Clay, I take a couple of ounces of liquid Bentonite clay and follow it with an 8-ounce glass of room temperature water. The room temperature water helps to expand the liquid Bentonite clay in the system, which will soak up the toxins within the body.

The Liquid Bentonite clay possesses a negative ionic electrical charge, which attracts positively charged particles in the form of toxic poisons and heavy metals. Because the toxins in the body are positively charged and the bentonite clay is negatively charged, they are attracted to one another like a magnet. So the bentonite clay will soak up the toxins and heavy metals and carry them out of your body through your stool.

I usually take a few ounces of the liquid bentonite clay with an 8-ounce glass of room temperature water and wait about an hour. I then take 2-4 capsules or 2 Tablespoons of psyllium husk with an 8-ounce glass of room temperature water. If you take the psyllium husk in powdered form, you must mix it into the water and drink it quickly, follow up with more water afterward. Make sure to drink the psyllium husk/water mixture within 30 seconds before it has time to thicken in the glass. I will take this method at various times throughout the day and right before bedtime. Wait at least an hour before or after eating prior to using the bentonite clay and/or psyllium husk or the vitamins and minerals from your food will not have time to assimilate within your body.

The Bentonite clay will soak up the toxins in the body and the psyllium husk is a fiber that will bind and carry the toxins out of your body the next time you experience a bowel movement. Ideally, you should be experiencing 2-3 bowel movements per day and you should not have to strain. If you are not experiencing 2-3 bowel movements per day, you are most likely constipated and dehydrated with toxic material in your colon and are in desperate need of a colon detox. I prefer using the yerba prima brand of liquid bentonite clay, as it doesn't have much of a taste at all and goes down quickly. I also use the yerba prima brand of psyllium husk, but most are all the same just make sure that the brand you choose doesn't have any fillers and the only ingredient should be ground psyllium husk.

If you enlist the detox kit method of detoxification, follow the instructions on the box. If you enlist the liquid Bentonite clay/Psyllium husk method, then you want to continue it for about a week or less depending upon your level of toxicity. If psyllium husk doesn't work well with your body, you can substitute 1-2 Tablespoons of freshly ground flaxseeds in a glass of water. Make sure to buy the flaxseeds whole and grind them fresh daily for the maximum effect. Flaxseeds which have already been ground prior to purchasing are already somewhat rancid and should not be consumed. It is important to pay attention to your body and how you feel when you do this cleanse. The kit is usually safer for those who are new to detoxification and it will help you ease into detoxification slower.

While conducting the colon cleanse, you may notice black, tarry stool, mucoid plaque, mucoid rope, slimy mucous, or parasites coming out of your body. Don't be alarmed as this is a normal part of detoxifying the colon and the first step into bringing your body back into balance. All of the sludge that has accumulated along your colon walls over the years will be eliminated and you will feel better once you are free from the toxic sludge that had taken up residence along your colon walls.

While conducting the colon cleanse, this is also a good time to cleanse the small intestines. Those with chronic illness or leaky gut may have a difficult time with the psyllium husk and find that it may not work for them or that their body cannot process the psyllium husk well. This was a problem I had when I had severe leaky gut. If someone has severe leaky gut, they will not be able to process much of anything they eat or drink. Therefore, this detox method may not work as well until after the gut lining is healed. Start by healing the gut lining first and also detoxify the small intestines with okra pepsin, which can help with healing the holes in the small intestines, thereby allowing the body to begin to work normally and you will be able to detoxify the body at that time. Okra Pepsin is made by Standard Process and can be purchased on Amazon.

Another good supplement to use for colon cleansing is called Triphala Gold made by Planetary Herbals; which is a combination of three different fruits native to India. Amla, Myrobalan, and Bellericmyrobalan are the three medicinal fruits that are found in Triphala. The benefits of Triphala include detoxification of the colon, contains antioxidants which boost the immune system, fights bacteria, normalizes cholesterol levels, helps fight cancer, improves respiratory function, improves digestive health by normalizing peristaltic function of the intestines, helps with asthma, improves eyesight, helps with weight loss, blood purifier, and helps to detoxify the liver. (10/11).

The side effects of Triphala is that you should not take it if you are blood thinning medication or pregnant. (10). Of course, you may experience a healing crisis when detoxifying the body and taking any type of supplement known to detoxify the body. So, you should expect symptoms of a healing crisis as explained in the chapter on Herxheimer reactions in this book.

Triphala comes in powder, tea, or capsules. I recommend the powder especially if you have leaky gut and are trying to improve digestive function whilst detoxifying the body. The capsules are also great for those who can assimilate capsules and to take with you when you travel.

To aid in detoxification of the small intestines, I prefer Okra Pepsin E3 by Standard Process. This works by using okra to bind to the toxic material attached in the small intestines which may be keeping you sick. If you have any type of brain fog that doesn't go away with a normal detox regimen, then the small intestines could be the issue and okra pepsin works well to clear debris in the small intestines.

Okra Pepsin can work quickly for some or it can take months to start working in others. I started with 3 capsules per day (1 in the morning, 1 at noon, and 1 at night) with a full glass of water for each. I took okra pepsin after each meal as it helped the body to digest the food I ate as well. Taking okra pepsin on an empty stomach can make your stomach burn, so always take it after a meal. It took over 2 months of taking the okra pepsin daily until I started seeing results with more white, slimy, stringy material coming out of my colon. The good news is that this also helped to get rid of my brain fog associated with the leaky gut and helped to heal the holes in the small intestines. The okra pepsin can eat away at the candida and/or parasites which may be attached to the walls of the small intestines. I truly believe that okra pepsin helped my digestive function and cleared my brain fog and I think this is a must for anyone with intestinal permeability issues.

A quick detox method for the colon is using activated charcoal. However, activated charcoal should only be used no more than 2 days a week. The activated charcoal capsules bind to the toxins in the colon and help to cart it out of the body. This will not scrub the colon of debris but it does seem to pick up a lot of the toxins residing in the colon. I have seen lots of yeast and parasites pass through using this method. Don't be alarmed if your stool is very black the next time you have a bowel movement. Also, taking too much activated charcoal can cause constipation issues, so make sure to drink plenty of water and take a couple of Triphala capsules to help move things along.

Another method of colon cleansing involves hydrotherapy, where you can visit a colon hydro therapist and have them perform the work of the colon cleanse for you. Some may not feel comfortable with someone doing a colonic for you; it can be stressful and uncomfortable. However, an experienced colon hydrotherapist can be extremely beneficial to your healing properly.

The colon cleanse should be done for 7 days and some may need to do it longer, but never more than two weeks at a time. If you opt for a kit, follow the instructions on the box for the length of time suggested on the kit. After you have successfully completed the colon cleanse, it is time to move onto cleansing the body of a fungus known as; Candida Albicans.

7

The Candida Cleanse

Candida Albicans, often referred to as just "Candida," is yeast like fungus that grows within the body and causes a host of health problems that manifests itself in various toxic symptoms. Candida is a common condition that approximately 85% of the population experiences, yet few know how to treat this underlying condition, which is a major root cause that may be causing their health symptoms.

Candida overgrowth can be caused from taking antibiotics, pharmaceutical drugs, birth control pills, sugar, refined carbohydrate foods, gluten, processed foods, long term illness and stress. All of these factors will alter the balance of good to bad bacteria in the body, creating an overgrowth of fungal yeast known as Candida Albicans.

Many people suffer from conditions like eczema, psoriasis, cancer, acne, headaches, sinusitis, PMS, hives, vaginal infections, infertility, fibromyalgia, allergies, sugar cravings, alcohol cravings, inability to lose weight, ringworm, bloating, gas, AIDS, HIV, Autism, ADHD, yeast infections, depression, insomnia, excessive mood swings, bad breath, thrush, thyroid problems, hormonal imbalance, learning disorders, autoimmune disease, Alzheimer's disease, Dementia, and many other conditions. If you experience any of these conditions listed above or any of the conditions listed in the "Symptoms of Toxicity" chart, it is highly likely that you have an overgrowth of Candida Albicans in your body. There is also a chronic form of Candida, which can be deadly if not treated properly, which is called Acetaldehyde (Auto Brewery Syndrome).

What is Acetaldehyde??? Acetaldehyde is a fungal waste product (1) that gives the hangover reaction or drunken feeling after eating a carbohydrate meal. Candida comes in many different forms and the acetaldehyde creates off-gassing at times. If you have a chronic candida, it can produce acetaldehyde, which can make you legally drunk just from eating certain foods while starving the candida. This condition had happened to me back in September of 2013, where I just came off a 15-day water fast and ate a plate of steamed vegetables and brown rice. I was at a conference where I was one of the speakers. After eating the vegetables and brown rice, I wasn't feeling so well and started to feel dizzy and nauseous, so I decided to head home early from the conference (I lived about an hour away).As I was in my car, my head started feeling funny and I started to "pass out" at the wheel. I felt like I was drunk, even though I had not consumed any alcohol in over a year. I had to open all the windows in the car for fresh air. For those who have ever been drunk in their lives, you know the feeling. That was very scary since I was driving on a freeway at the time, during rush hour traffic, and it took every ounce of strength to make it home safely.

I had already known that I had a candida problem, but to have acetaldehyde means that a form of candida yeast (brewer's yeast) is in the bloodstream and will produce the effects of being drunk even though you have not had any alcohol to drink. It is an off-gassing effect of the candida fungus which turns into pure alcohol in the presence of carbohydrate meals. (15). When you have a chronic candida infection in the bloodstream, it is like having a brewery within your body, turning the yeast into pure alcohol in the presence of carbohydrate meals. This effect happened to me a few more times throughout September and October of 2013 before I was finally able to reverse it naturally. I had been tested for food allergies, but the test also revealed measurable amounts of brewer's yeast in my bloodstream, which had caused the auto brewery syndrome I had experienced on multiple occasions in 2013.

In order to properly detoxify your body from candida and be on the road to good health, you must have completed the colon cleanse first to clear the channels of elimination. It is wise to change your eating habits to starve the candida of its fuel source while on the candida cleanse to achieve maximum efficiency. If you do not change your eating habits, you will continue to feed the candida and you will not be able to eradicate it from your body.

There are plenty of candida detox kits on the market that will help to eliminate candida. All of the detox kits will work differently depending upon the severity of the candida. Some people will have good luck with a candida kit if their candida isn't too severe of a problem. However, some people experience systemic/chronic candida or the candida has reached the bloodstream, which are severe types of candida infection that are difficult to eradicate with just a candida kit, in which case you will need a more detailed detoxification regimen. Here are a few of the Candida supplements I have tried over the years that work to eradicate Candida in the body.

Anti-Fungal Treatments:

Diflucan: a doctor's prescription is needed for this medication and Diflucan is a medication which can harm the liver with prolonged use. It is not suggested to take this product for more 3 days. According to Ann Boroch; CNC, the Diflucan should only be for a jumpstart of three 150 mg tablets where you take 1 pill every three days for one week.

I was at the point in my health where nothing was working for me and I finally had to ask a doctor to prescribe this for me and then some nystatin afterward. Diflucan is a last resort and is suited for those with cancer, autoimmune disease or mental illness. (9).

If you decide to jump start your program with Diflucan; you need to make sure your doctor is knowledgeable enough to be monitoring your liver enzymes during this process. You also don't want to take Diflucan for long periods of time due to the toxic effect upon your liver.

Nystatin: Nystatin is another anti-fungal prescribed medication which has less of a toxic effect upon your liver. However, Nystatin will take months to be able to get into the bloodstream to have any positive effect upon a severe candida infection and most doctors aren't knowledgeable about Candida and don't prescribe Nystatin for much longer than 30 days, which is completely pointless. After the Nystatin prescription runs out, you may need to switch to herbal antifungals for biofilms (see the biofilm chapter).

Make sure to meet with a doctor who is knowledgeable about systemic candida infections and can help you to heal. I was never lucky enough to find such a doctor, even after seeing multiple NDs, integrative MDs, DCs, and finally had to figure it out on my own to heal myself once the Nystatin ran out.

Tanalbit by Intensive Nutrition Inc.: Tanalbit is another over the counter supplement which can help to get rid of candida overgrowth that can be affecting your digestion. This is a very strong formula made from lotus rhizome root extract and zinc tannate. The rhizome root extracts targets candida biofilm, yeast and bacteria within the digestive tract. Excellent for those with intestinal permeability issues which may be caused by yeast. Take this very slowly with a smaller dosage and work your way up to the dosage on the bottle.

The zinc tannates in Tanalbit are an astringent that helps to get rid of bacteria and fungus. If you have chronic candida, the type that creates acetaldehyde (auto brewery syndrome) within the body, you will find that the Tanalbit is very strong and this will give you a massive healing crisis. Go slow with the dosage to not overwhelm your liver of too many toxins being dumped at once.

The other issue with Tanalbit is that it contains high heat milk powder which can be problematic for those with dairy allergies and lactose intolerances. Otherwise, this does work well but you will definitely feel the effects if you have a chronic candida condition. If you do not have chronic candida, the Tanalbit will not give you a healing crisis.

Candex by Pure Essence Labs: this formula helps to digest fungal cell walls, which is the biofilm barrier protecting the candida.

CandidaEx by Universal Formulas: this is also a strong formula, which does contain a couple of ingredients which help to break through the biofilm of the candida. This formula contains such herbs as cat's claw, olive leaf extract, goldenseal root, undedylenic acid, grapefruit seed extract, Oregon grape root, and many more herbs.

Oregano Oil: Oregano Oil is an anti-bacterial, anti-fungal, anti-parasitic, and anti-viral agent. Oregano's antifungal properties are used to treat chronic candidiasis and inhibit the growth of Candida Albicans. (11). "The antimicrobial and antifungal properties of oregano are attributed to thymol and carvacrol. Clinical studies have shown oregano to be extremely effective in inhibiting the growth of Candida albicans. Additional clinical studies demonstrate that oregano oil has anti-microbial properties against a large array of bacteria including Escherichia coli, Klebsiella pneumoniae, Salmonella enterica and Staphylococcus aureus." (11).

It is imperative to use only pure wild Oregano Oil. Many oregano oils are standardized, which means they are processed with chemical agents. Make sure that the wild oregano oil is not standardized and contains at least 70% carvacrol and thymol. I use North American Herb and Spice Oregano oil and oreganol extra strength capsules. Also, Oregamax and Oregano Oil juice by the same company.

It may take years of using Oregano Oil daily to be able to get the results you are seeking. I took oregano oil for a period of over 2 years to finally get control of the systemic candida infection in my gut. I used 1 dropperful of Oregano oil down my throat; 3-5 times per day. I also used a few drops of Oregano oil under my tongue 3-5 times daily; I did this at the same time of the dropperful down my throat. Be advised that Oregano Oil is very spicy hot and you need to drink a full glass of water following your dosage to get rid of the burning feeling in your mouth. If you find the oil too harsh, there are "enteric coated capsules to ensure the tablets pass through the stomach and disintegrate in the intestines." (11).

Pau d Arco: Also known as Lapacho or Taheebo, but more commonly referred to as Pau d' Arco, these trees are native to South America. Pau d' Arco comes mainly in the form of a tea or drops. However, "The herbal tea form of pau d'arco remedy is ineffective due to the insolubility of the naphthaquinone active constituents in water - therefore the remedy cannot be used in the form of a tea. However, the pau d'arco can be taken in the form of herbal capsules or tablets and these are widely available, each providing 300 mg of powdered bark for remedial action against various conditions." (13). Truthfully, the tea tastes horrible, so I would rather take the drops in a glass of water quickly.

Pau d Arco is an antibacterial, anti-viral, anti-parasitic, anti-fungal, and anti-inflammatory which is effective against gastrointestinal candidiasis, ringworm, herpes virus, cancer particularly leukemia, AIDS, parasites, and many other bacterial, viral, and fungal infections. (13).

Grapefruit Seed Extract: "Grapefruit Seed Extract (GSE) has been used for killing a wide variety of bacteria (such as: Salmonella, E. Coli, Staph and Strep germs), viruses, herpes, parasites, and fungi, including Candida. It is effective against more than 800 bacterial and viral strains, 100 strains of fungus, as well as a large number of single-cell and multi-celled parasites. It has also proven to be effective against food poisoning and diarrhea." (12). It is also non-toxic and has no harmful side effects, although it tastes very bitter. I prefer the Nutribiotic brand of Grapefruit Seed Extract and I put the drops directly into a few ounces of water and drink it down very quickly. "GSE is able to discriminate between the harmful bacteria and the healthy bacteria. In fact, GSE can actually encourage the growth of beneficial bacteria by inhibiting the growth of destructive microbes." (12).

Caprylic Acid: "Caprylic acid belongs to a class of medium-chain saturated fatty acids. Found naturally in dairy products, palm oil, and coconut oil." (14). Caprylic acid is anti-bacterial, anti-viral and anti-fungal, which can help with candida yeast. It is also said to treat ringworm, high cholesterol levels, Crohn's disease, intestinal candidiasis and high blood pressure. I have used the brand Caproyl which contains 1,600 mg of caprylic acid per Tablespoon.

Thorne Research Formula SF722: Includes 10-Undecenoic Acid and is very effective against hard to tackle Candida infections. This worked great for me, in conjunction with biofilm disruptors discussed in the following chapter on biofilms.

DIDA Clear: This formula combines deodorized garlic, barberry powder, caprylic acid, undecylenic acid, grapefruit extract and lactobacillus acidophilus so you get all of the benefits of various anti fungals in one formula. This product is made from vitacost.

Oregon Grape: Oregon grape shares much of the same benefits of goldenseal as they both contain Berberine, which is an anti-fungal to control candida. "Oregon grape root contains berberine, also found in barberry, coptis, and goldenseal. The herb also contains phytochemicals with similar activity, including columbamine, hydrastine, jatrorrhizine, oxyacanthine, and tetrahydroberberine, as well as tannins." (18). "It is also traditionally used as a bitter tonic to stimulate digestion and externally for its antimicrobial properties. The active constituents in Oregon grape root have shown substantial antimicrobial and antifungal activity in vitro, though these activities are unproven in human trials." (18).

Oregon grape has a high level of berberine and Vitamin C and works as an antibiotic, an astringent, alterative, diuretic and it works well as a laxative. It has the ability to stimulate a thyroid, which makes it a good option for those that have an inactive or under producing thyroid. It is helpful in treating fevers, upset stomachs, scurvy, reduces sore throats and boosts the immune system. (19).

It can also be used topically to treat acne, abrasions, eczema, psoriasis and similar conditions. To use it topically, a small dab of the Oregon grape root extract is applied to the area. (19).

Goldenseal: Goldenseal is an herbal antibiotic, anti-inflammatory, astringent, and immune system enhancer. "Goldenseal contains calcium, iron, manganese, vitamin A, vitamin C, vitamin E, B-complex, and other nutrients and minerals." (20). The primary alkaloid in Goldenseal is Berberine which is why it is effective against bacteria, protozoa, fungi, Streptococci, anti-bacterial, and anti-fungal. (20).

It has been used as a medication for inflammatory conditions; such as respiratory, digestive and genito-urinary tract inflammation induced by allergy or infection. (20). "It soothes irritated mucus membranes helping the eyes, ears, nose and throat. Goldenseal works for respiratory problems, colds or flu, when taken at the first sign of these issues. It has also been used to help reduce fevers, and relieve congestion and excess mucous." (20).

"Goldenseal cleanses and promotes healthy glandular functions by increasing bile flow and digestive enzymes, therefore regulating healthy liver and spleen functions. It can relieve constipation and may also be used to treat infections of the bladder and intestines as well as help with allergic rhinitis, hay fever, laryngitis, hepatitis, cystitis, and alcoholic liver disease, eczema, ringworm, excessive menstruation, internal bleeding, wounds, earaches, gum infections, sore throat, boils, abscesses, and carbuncles." (20). Goldenseal can also be used as a wash, drops, and a poultice for multiple uses mentioned above.

Olive Leaf: Olive leaf is an anti-bacterial, anti-fungal, anti-viral, and anti- parasitic. "In the early 1900s scientists isolated a bitter compound called oleuropein from olive leaf that was thought to give the olive tree its disease resistance. Oleuropein inhibited the growth of viruses, bacteria, fungi and parasites. Olive leaf can help to treat influenza, the common cold, candida infections, meningitis, Epstein-Barr virus (EBV), encephalitis, herpes I and II, human herpes virus 6 and 7, shingles (Herpes zoster), HIV/ARC/AIDS, chronic fatigue, hepatitis B, pneumonia, tuberculosis, gonorrhea, malaria, dengue, severe diarrhea, and dental, ear, urinary tract and surgical infections." (16).

Olive leaf has many health benefits aside from being an anti-fungal. It works for "stabilizing blood sugar levels, parasites (giardia, intestinal worms, malaria forming protozoa, microscopic protozoa, pinworms, ringworm, roundworm, tapeworms), boosting immune function, fighting infection, increasing resistance to disease, lowering blood pressure, anthrax, arteriosclerosis, arthritis, autoimmune disorders, barium chloride and calcium induced arrhythmia, boosts energy levels, brain and nervous conditions, candida, cardiovascular conditions, chest complaints, chlamydia, chronic fatigue, chronic joint ache, chronic toenail fungus infection, colds & flu, cold sores, dengue, dental, ear, urinary tract and surgical infections, dissolves cholesterol, encephalitis, Epstein-Barr virus (EBV), fevers, fibromyalgia, gastric ulcers caused by H. pylori, gastrointestinal conditions, genital herpes, genital warts, gonorrhea, hemorrhoid pain-relief, hepatitis A, B, C, herpes I and II, HIV/ARC/AIDS, human herpes virus 6 and 7, improves blood flow, improves symptoms of chronic fatigue syndrome and related conditions, increases bile secretions, lupus, malaria, meningitis (bacterial/viral), mononucleosis, nervous tension, normalization of heart beat irregularities, pneumonia, psoriasis, rabies, respiratory conditions, rheumatic fever, salmonella, severe diarrhea, shingles (Herpes zoster), sinus infections, soothes mucous membranes, staphylococcal food poisoning, streptococcus infection in throat, syphilis, toothache, toxic shock syndrome, trichinosis, tuberculosis, vaginitis, vasodilator effect on the smooth layer of coronary arteries, warts." (16).

Anti-Fungal Foods:

Various foods contain anti-fungal compounds which help to get rid of candida naturally. These foods are to be used in conjunction with a combination of herbal antibiotics mentioned above. The anti-fungal foods consist of garlic, leeks, onions, ginger root, grapefruit seed extract, oregano, black walnut, and Pau D'arco. I personally like to use a clove of garlic, a hunk of ginger, 1 Tablespoon of Olive Oil, and 1 cup of Water all blended together with a hand-held stick type blender and taken at night before bed. Another way to rid the body of candida is to make sure to include anti-fungal foods to your diet on a daily basis, use lots of garlic, onions, and oregano in your cooking.

It is also imperative to re-populate your body of the good bacteria. When you have candida, the bad bacteria in your body outweigh the good bacteria, which is another factor that is keeping you sick. Adding probiotics and prebiotics to your diet will also help to starve the candida from your body and balance the ratio of good bacteria to bad bacteria. Do not take the garlic/ginger mixture, candida detox kit, or any candida medication (herbal or prescription) within 3 hours of probiotics or prebiotics to experience the best results for eradicating Candida. This is why I take the garlic/ginger mixture at night and then do the probiotics and prebiotics during the day and stop 3 hours before taking the garlic/ginger mixture.

If you have systemic candida, you may notice that even though you may be eating a perfect diet that you are still having health problems. For systemic candida infections, it may take years to finally get your body back into balance and rid yourself of candida. Be diligent with the candida diet, anti fungals, probiotics, and healing supplements (glutamine, aloe vera, turmeric).

Oregano Oil Enema:

You can also add a few drops of Oregano Oil to an enema bag of water or to your coffee enemas to kill any parasites and fungal infections within the colon. You would do this prior to ever starting the probiotic retention enemas. I have found that this method helps to dislodge a lot of the fungus attached to the colon walls. I noticed a lot of fungus and whitish stringy material dislodging from my colon when I completed an oregano oil enema.

Make sure to also re-populate the colon with probiotics a few hours after doing an oregano oil enema. Natren probiotics are powdered probiotics which can easily be added to an enema bag with water and used as a retention enema. A retention enema is when you hold the enema for a period, which can be 15 minutes up to a few hours. For those with dairy allergies, Natren probiotics also has a non-dairy version. You can find the complete probiotic enema in the earlier chapter on healing leaky gut.

Foods you cannot eat on a candida diet or while detoxing from cancer; no sugars, no starches, no processed foods, no high fructose corn syrup, no fruit, no dried fruit, no melons, no artificial sweeteners, no sodas, no fermented foods, no malted products, no alcoholic beverages, no yeasts, no breads, no cheeses, no vinegar containing foods or condiments, no gluten, and no antibiotics.

I have outlined a list of foods that you can eat while on the candida diet. It is good to stick to this list while you have any illness as well, because fungus; such as, Candida Albicans, can also fuel cancer growth, inflammation, and chronic illness. So, by eating these foods, you can aid in eliminating candida and help to eradicate many health conditions.

Foods Allowed on the Candida Diet:

Vegetables: asparagus, avocado, broccoli, brussels sprouts, cabbage, cauliflower, celery, cucumber, collard greens, eggplant, garlic (raw), green beans, kale, leeks, okra, onions, peppers, radish, seaweed,

spaghetti squash, spinach, romaine, summer squash, swiss chard, tomatoes, turnip, and zucchini.

- Vegetables starve the Candida of the sugar and mold that feed it.
- Vegetables can absorb fungal poisons and carry them out of your body.
- Avoid starchy vegetables such as carrots, sweet potatoes, potatoes, yams, corn, butternut squash, beets, peas, parsnips and all beans except green beans.
- Buy your vegetables fresh and eat them raw, steam or grill them. Add a little garlic and onions for flavor as they are especially helpful with Candida.
- If you steam the veggies, drink the water that is left over, it contains most of the potassium and B vitamins that are leached from the veggies when they are cooked.
- Eat at least 5-9 servings of vegetables everyday (a serving is ½ a cup). Thus, eat 2-5 cups a day.
- Do not use any dressings on salads aside from fresh lemon juice and extra virgin olive oil.

Live Yogurt Cultures: plain yogurt, probiotics.

- Live yogurt cultures (or probiotics) help your gut to repopulate itself with good bacteria.
- The live bacteria in the yogurt will crowd out the Candida yeast and restore balance to your system.
- Buy only plain yogurt that is Rbgh/Rbst free. Greek yogurt is a good choice, without any additives.
- Yogurt from goat and sheep milk is even better, as they tend to contain fewer chemicals and goats and sheep's milk are easier to digest than cow's milk.
- Good bacteria will also produce antifungal enzymes that can help you fight Candida.

Proteins: beef, chicken, wild fish, eggs, shrimp.

- Proteins are almost completely free of sugars and mold, so they restrict the Candida.
- Eat only fresh, grass fed, organic meat.
- Eat only wild caught salmon, cod, swordfish, sardines, and trout. No farmed fish or Atlantic salmon.
- Processed meat like lunch meat, bacon, smoked, vacuum packed, and spam, is loaded with dextrose, nitrates, sulphates, and sugars and should never be consumed.

Nuts and Seeds: almonds, walnuts, cashews, pecans, filberts, brazil, pumpkin seeds, and sunflower seeds.

- Nuts and seeds are a high protein food that starves candida and restricts its growth.
- Avoid peanuts and pistachios as they tend to have higher mold content and the peanut is not a nut, but a legume.
- You can remove mold by soaking the nuts in water. Make sure the nuts and seeds are raw.
- You can also buy pure nut butters, such as cashew and almond butter.

Gluten Free Grains: buckwheat, millet, amaranth, quinoa, wild rice, and brown rice.

- Grains contain a high amount of fiber, excellent for keeping the colon clear.
- Grains also act like a pipe cleaner in your intestine, grabbing nasty toxins; such as, pollutants, chemicals, pesticides and heavy metals.
- Make sure any grain is gluten free.

Herbs and Spices: basil, black pepper, cayenne, cilantro, cinnamon, cloves, cumin, curry, dill, garlic, ginger, nutmeg, oregano, paprika, rosemary, tarragon, thyme, and turmeric.

- Contains antioxidants and anti-fungal properties.
- Increases circulation and reduces inflammation.
- Improves digestion and alleviates constipation.
- Most herbs and spices are beneficial in your fight against candida.
- Great for livening up food on a limited candida diet.

Oils: virgin coconut oil, olive oil, sesame oil, pumpkin seed oil, macadamia nut oil, almond oil, flax oil, safflower oil, sunflower oil, coconut butter, ghee, and grass-fed butter.

- Use cold pressed oils and virgin oils.
- Heating or boiling destroys many of the oils' nutrients.
- Only virgin coconut oil or ghee should be used for cooking because it retains its nutrients at high heats.
- All other oils are great on salads or drizzled over vegetables.

Beverages: lemon water, cinnamon tea, green tea, clove tea, ginger tea, chamomile tea, pau d' arco tea, peppermint tea, licorice tea, fennel tea, lemongrass tea, dandelion tea.

- Many herbal teas have anti-fungal properties.

- If you're missing your morning coffee, try green Tea, black tea or Teecino offers a dandelion beverage to replace coffee (caffeine free and gluten free available).
- If caffeine free: use herbal teas or Teecino herbal beverage.
- Adding lemon to the water helps to alkalize the body.

The candida cleanse can be performed at the same time as the parasite cleanse, which is discussed next, although if the candida is systemic than you may want to only target the candida first because the die-off symptoms of chronic candida are very harsh and should be taken very slowly to not overwhelm the liver with too many toxins at once.

Many times, if Candida cannot be eradicated using these methods, it can be due to the acetaldehyde and biofilm formations. If you find that you are still chronically ill after conducting the candida cleanse, it can be due to biofilms. I will discuss biofilms in a later chapter and how to safely eradicate the biofilm formations so you can eradicate the chronic/systemic candida infection. If you have a chronic disease, chances are good that there is a biofilm formation as the root cause.

It is also wise to vary the anti-fungals to see which one may work for you. Some of you may be fortunate and can use a candida detox kit once and feel better. For others, you may have to take the individual anti-fungals for years to get a handle on the candida fungal infection.

I personally had to resort to the Diflucan for 3 days, then Nystatin, then herbal anti-fungals and biofilm disruptors to finally get a handle on my chronic candida infection in my body and bloodstream. It took many years as I was also dealing with the severe leaky gut so many of the anti-fungals weren't working properly on my system because they weren't being absorbed.

Once you have gotten a better handle on the candida infection, you can target the parasites within your body. As I have said before, you can do both the candida and the parasite cleanses at the same time if the die-off or Herxheimer reactions aren't too great, otherwise only do the candida cleanse first and then the parasite cleanse afterward.

8

Those Nasty Parasites

"Millions of Americans develop parasitic infections and symptoms often go unnoticed or are misdiagnosed. These microscopic creatures are typically picked up through food and water. An infection can lead to serious health problems, including seizures, blindness, pregnancy complications, heart failure and even death." (20).

You may have parasites if you live with animals, have eaten improperly cooked foods (i.e.; sushi), drank water from an unclean source, or have eaten any vegetables that weren't cleaned properly. If you suspect you may have parasites, you can do a parasite cleanse to rid your body of the nasty critters. Even if you aren't sure you have parasites, it is still a good idea to do a parasite cleanse just in case, you may be surprised at what comes out.

Symptoms of parasitic infections include; teeth grinding at night, being diagnosed with iron deficiency anemia, skin irritations, hives, rashes, eczema, Rosacea, pain or aching in muscles and joints, sleep disturbances, never feeling full after meals, constipation, gas, diarrhea, IBS, nervousness, chronic fatigue, reddened eyes, itchy anus and depressed immune function just to name a few. (19).

Many people never realize that parasites may be living within their body and creating their health problems. Parasites consist of whipworms, roundworms, tapeworms, hookworms, ropeworms, flukes, and many other nasty invaders of the body which may create a myriad of the health problems you may be experiencing.

Parasites are made up of proteins that can usually be eliminated through the digestive enzymes that are produced naturally within your digestive system. However, if you are low on hydrochloric acid or digestive enzymes; which digest proteins, then the parasites can attach themselves to your intestines and begin feeding off of your food supply. Parasites also attach to your system when your immunity is lowered due to chronic infections or illness. Parasitic infestation causes a nutrient deficiency within the host (you) and eventually may lead to many chronic illnesses. Parasites live off of the host and feed off of the host. Therefore, the parasite gets stronger and multiplies within the host and the host can get weaker because their nutrient supply is being diminished and the nutrients are eaten by the parasite.

Even when doing a parasite cleanse, it is important to cleanse for parasites for at least six weeks straight and then take a break. The parasite cleanses will need to be rotated and repeated so the parasites don't become immune to any of the anti-parasitic herbal concoctions, which happens often.

Common Types of Parasites:

"The two main types of intestinal parasites are helminths and protozoa. Helminths are worms with many cells. Tapeworms, pinworms, and roundworms are among the most common helminths in the United States. In their adult form, helminths cannot multiply in the human body. Protozoa have only one cell, and can multiply inside the human body, which can allow serious infections to develop. Intestinal parasites are usually transmitted when someone comes in contact with infected feces (for example, through contaminated soil, food, or water). In the U.S., the most common protozoa are giardia and cryptosporidium." (16).

This is a brief list of several types of Helminths and Protozoan parasites, which are commonly found in humans and animals. These parasites are transmitted through soil, water or food. There are four main types of helminthic parasites consisting of nematodes, cestodes, trematodes, and monogeneans. (1). The most common protozoa are Giardia and Cryptosporidium. (16).

84

HELMINTHS:

Roundworms (nematodes): The nematode species of worms contains hookworms, whipworms, roundworms, pinworms, threadworms, and trichinosis. The eggs are eaten with contaminated food, which end up infesting the host. The roundworm can grow up to 1 meter in length, which is 39.5 inches approximately. "Intestinal roundworm infections constitute the largest group of helminthic diseases in humans." (7).

Symptoms of a nematode infection may include blood in the stool, cough, trouble breathing (lung issues), skin infections, river blindness, pneumonia, wheezing, asthma, abdominal pain, diarrhea, constipation, vomiting, fever, edema, facial edema, rashes, encephalitis, rashes, pain upon swallowing, inflammation, abscesses, lymphedema, dermatitis, glaucoma, urticaria, worm protrusion from the skin, anal itching (frequently at night), and allergic reactions just to name a few.

Due to the many symptoms of a nematode infection, parasitic infections can be the root cause of many diseases; such as, Crohn's disease, pancreatitis, lymphedema, Asthma, Hodgkin's Lymphoma, appendicitis, diverticulitis, Lupus, Leprosy, Tuberculosis, Anemia, Cardiac insufficiency, and more. (7).

These types of parasitic infection are often passed in undercooked meats, water supply, and feces. So, it is imperative to cook all meats properly to a temperature of 140 degrees, boil water especially if traveling abroad, and always wash your hands after using the toilet.

Tapeworms (cestodes): a cestode is an intestinal tape worm, that looks like a huge layer of tape, which attaches to the intestines and sucks up all nutrients and food in the body. This usually causes the host to lose considerable amounts of weight because they are not getting any nutrients and the tapeworm is getting it all.

Tapeworms are usually contracted through contaminated foods and undercooked meats from an infected animal. (6). They can also be passed through an infected human who goes to the restroom without wiping properly and doesn't wash their hands and then proceeds to prepare a meal. (6). If the tapeworm cannot be detected through stool testing, which is very common as stool testing isn't very reliable to detect parasitic infection, the doctor can test for parasites using a blood test for antibodies, a computed tomography (CT) scan or a magnetic resonance imaging (MRI) scan for more serious infections. (6).

Flukes (trematodes): Trematodes; also called Flukes, contain suckers and pierce holes in the organs which they attach too, which then suck the nutrients out of the host. The various types of flukes are lung flukes, liver flukes, intestinal flukes, pancreatic flukes, eye flukes, and blood flukes. (8).

Flukes are invading 300 million people per year and are most common in Asian countries but are increasing in numbers in the United States. (9). An adult liver fluke can produce over 25,000 eggs per day and lead to such symptoms as; vomiting, diarrhea, fever, stomach aches, increased white blood cell count, intestinal blocking, muscle aches and pains. (9).

If you are infected with Flukes, it is highly likely that you will receive various diagnoses; such as, pancreatitis, cystitis, Hepatitis A, Hepatitis B, Hepatitis C, Hepatitis D, Hepatitis E, Viral Hepatitis, Inflammatory Bowel Disease, Typhoid Fever, Tuberculosis, and Urinary Tract Infection (8). Liver flukes are very common in Cancer patients with Liver cancer, but can also be found in all types of cancer (10). Flukes are also responsible for Cystic Fibrosis, Down's syndrome and Polycystic Kidney Disease (10), which is genetic in nature.

Flukes can be contracted through eating watercress, water chestnuts, other water plants, raw fish, raw crabs, raw crayfish, and fresh water snails (11). This may be why fluke infestation is more prevalent in Asian countries as these types of foods are staples of Asian cuisine, although the fluke infestation is increasing in numbers in the United States. To avoid fluke infestation, wash all vegetables very well and cook fish properly.

Ropeworms (monogeneans): "Rope parasites can attach to intestinal walls with suction bubbles, which later develop into suction heads. Walls of the rope parasites consist of scale-like cells forming multiple branched channels along the parasite's length. Rope parasites can move by jet propulsion, passing gas bubbles through these channels. Currently known anthelmintic methods include special enemas. Most humans are likely hosting these helminths."

Rope worms release toxins in the intestinal tract and bloodstream which diminish the immunity of the host. When rope worms are released, usually during an enema or an effective parasite cleanse, it will look like the inside of the intestines, very slimy and rope like. For this reason, many rope worms aren't realized because they are passed off as a part of the detoxification process where strings of slime are passed through the colon due to colon detoxification and enemas.

One way to distinguish the rope worm is too pay close attention to what you are expelling into the toilet, even though something may look like slimy mucous coming from your bowels, it may actually be a rope worm.

PROTOZOA:

Giardia: this is a protozoa regarded as the most common intestinal parasite infecting humans and is transmitted through food, water or soil that has been contaminated with feces from an infected human or animal. (17).

Symptoms of a Giardia infection include diarrhea, gas, greasy floating stools, upset stomach, nausea, vomiting, dehydration, stomach/abdominal cramps, itchy skin, hives, swelling of eye & joints. (17).

Cryptosporidium: often referred to as "Crypto," which can be passed through food, water, or soil that has been contaminated with feces from an infected human or animal. (18).

Symptoms of a Crypto infection include watery diarrhea, nausea, fever, vomiting, dehydration, and/or stomach cramps or pain. (18). Many will show no symptoms of infection at all.

Parasite Cleanse:

The parasite cleanse can be done in conjunction with the candida cleanse, but it depends upon how advanced your candida or parasitic infections are to determine whether you should do them together or separate. A lot of toxins may be released when killing off parasites, so depending upon your level of infection, you may want to do this cleanse separately and after the Candida cleanse.

You will need the following ingredients; Wormwood Capsules, Clove Capsules, Black Walnut tincture or capsules, Neem capsules, Proteolytic enzymes (Doctor's Best, see my favorites section in the appendix). The cloves will kill the eggs and larvae of the parasites, while the Wormwood and Black walnut kills the adult parasites. Neem also is anti-parasitic and a great addition to the parasite cleanse. The digestive enzymes help to digest the protein of the parasite. If you also have pets, you will need to add in food grade diatomaceous earth for your pets at the same time you are conducting a parasite cleanse.

A method in conjunction with the parasite cleanse is to take Proteolytic (protease) enzymes that digests proteins because the parasite is made up of protein and taking the enzymes will help to digest the parasite and release it from the intestines and colon. The wormwood, cloves, black walnut, and Neem can also kill the parasites but may not work on all types of parasites or the parasite becomes adapted to the treatment. The combination of the four can at least reduce the strength of the parasites, letting them be eaten and released by the protease (protein digesting) enzymes.

The method of the parasite cleanse is to take 3 of the Wormwood capsules and 3 of the Clove capsules, 3 times a day for up to six weeks. That is a total of 9 clove capsules per day and 9 wormwood capsules per day. At the same time; take 20 drops of the Black Walnut tincture, mixed in water, 3 times a day for up to six weeks. That is a total of 60 drops of black walnut tincture per day. The black walnut tincture will also help to eradicate candida within the body as well as the parasites. There is also a capsule of wormwood combination that includes the cloves, black walnut and wormwood together. There is also a black walnut capsule as opposed to the tincture. In which case, follow the directions on the bottle. With the Neem capsules, I was taking 2 capsules, 3 times per day in conjunction with the wormwood, black walnut, cloves and digestive enzymes.

I have also used the black walnut, clove, and wormwood drops and added about 2 dropperfuls to a coffee enema to kill any parasites that are in the anus. I have done this when I had extreme anal itching at night, which kept me awake for hours. To relieve the itch, I did an enema of this mixture and immediately heard bubbling in the anus area. When I expelled the enema contents, there was a ball of yeast that came out with it. Whether any parasites were in that ball of yeast is unknown, but I could sleep soundly the rest of the night with no more anal itching or feeling like worms were crawling around inside of my anus. It is probably a good idea to follow this up with a probiotic enema to re-populate the good bacteria within the colon.

It is also imperative to increase the plant enzymes within your body while you are doing the parasite cleanse above. The parasite cleanse can help to weaken and kill off the parasites and the protease enzymes can also help to eradicate the parasites. It is a one-two punch for parasitic control. The plant enzymes are the Proteolytic enzymes which dissolve protein. A plant enzyme formula should contain protease, which digests proteins. Proteolytic enzymes or proteases can also be plant based which digest proteins; the plants used to digest proteins are pineapple and papaya. Bromelain is in the core of pineapple and Papain is found in papaya. Both of these will also digest proteins. This is the main ingredient to be able to digest the protein of the parasites. At least 285,000 HUT of protease is needed per day. HUT stands for hemoglobin units on tyrosine basis, which measures hydrolyzing proteins into peptides and amino acids. Find a plant based digestive enzyme with a high amount of protease HUT units to help to digest the parasites. The best one I have found is from Doctor's Best, which contains 95,000 HUT per capsule.

An experiment I conducted on myself was to do 4 wormwood capsules, 4 black walnut, 2 clove capsules, and 10 digestive enzymes with a protease HUT level of 950,000 (I did this 3 times per day before meals for only 3 days). What I found was amazing, my face increased in redness and bumpy appearance at the site of the Rosacea near my nose. The open sores near my lips became more inflamed and reddened. There would also be a lot of foul smelling gas as the protease ate away at the proteins (parasites) in my intestines. This is too much of a dosage to continue for six weeks, but on occasion it is good to switch up the dosage and kill more parasites that have already become immune to the normal dosage.

Parasites are elusive, they become accustomed to various treatments over time and can continue to thrive, even though you may be doing a parasite cleanse and eating properly. For this reason, it is imperative to vary the parasite treatments and dosages so the parasites do not get accustomed to one treatment. So, one day I would do 2 clove capsules, 2 wormwood capsules, 2 black walnut capsules, 2 Artemisia combination capsules by nature's sunshine, 2 digestive enzyme capsules by Doctors Best (protease HUT of 95,000 per capsule). I would also take a teaspoon to 1 Tablespoon of food grade diatomaceous earth mixed in water at night. Now to vary this, I would also sometimes add in Neem capsules to the daily regime. I would then vary this dosage daily so the parasites wouldn't get used to a specific dosage and become immune.

With varying the dosage, I would notice that I would occasionally release more parasites. Some days I would stop all treatment except for the digestive enzymes before meals, and then I would feel an itching at my anal area between 1:00 am-3:00 am, which woke me up, and I wouldn't be able to go back to sleep until after 3:00 am when the parasites settled down and then I would wake up again at 6:00 am and take a larger dosage of the parasite formula of wormwood, clove, black walnut, Neem, and digestive enzymes. You can experiment with the dosages yourself to find what works best for you, but vary the dosages on occasion so the parasites do not become immune.

Whenever I felt itching at night and took the parasite cleanse in the morning, I would pass a parasite with my stool. After having a bowel movement, I would do a coffee enema with black walnut tincture, clove tincture, and garlic oil. This is another key to releasing parasites is through the daily enemas. I prefer coffee enemas because it cleanses the liver for any toxins and liver flukes and it also can cleanse the colon. When using coffee enemas, it is difficult to see if any parasites have released from the body due to the color of the coffee. You will find information on the coffee enema in the liver cleansing chapter. You can also choose to do a water cleansing enema or go get a colon hydrotherapist to do this for you. When you are doing the enema, you should be massaging the entire length of your small intestines and large intestines.

When I am holding the water or coffee from the enema in my colon, I will massage starting from the left side of my colon and massaging up the intestines and under the breast bone across to the other side of the intestines and down to the colon. What you may notice with the intestinal massage is that you may experience tender spots along the length of the intestines. It is important to massage these tender areas until whatever is causing the pain and discomfort moves further down the intestines to be finally released into the large intestines and colon. Sometimes these "tender spots" can be a nest of parasites holding on with suction cup strength, so massaging these areas may release the nest of parasites.

I have personally felt tender spots on my left side of the intestines below my left breast and then the tender spot moved toward my right side of the intestines and I would keep massaging until I felt no more tender areas along my intestines. Whatever could be lodged in the intestinal area would be released with the intestinal massage. This takes patience as it can take many years of consistent massage, enemas, and parasite cleansing to release the parasites from your system. The amount of time it takes is directly correlated with the degree of parasitic infestation.

Parasitic infestation is difficult to measure because the traditional tests for parasites are inconclusive and inaccurate because they are only testing for a few species of parasites, not all of them. So, you could test negative for parasites with a typical comprehensive stool test but you could still have parasites. This is what happened to me, I had tested positive for parasites in my blood using a live blood scan analysis, but then tested negative for parasites using a comprehensive stool analysis with parasitology. Although I tested negative, I still had worms coming out of my stool and felt the worms crawling around my anal cavity at night.

A good indication that you may have parasites is you will sometimes feel anal itching in the middle of the night. Parasites are most active at night and that is when you may be awoken feeling the itching in the anal area. It is important not to scratch because you can carry the eggs or the parasites underneath your nails. I often had this symptom, but then it became more sporadic where sometimes I would feel the parasites being active at night and other nights I wouldn't.

There is a theory of the moon phases and parasitic activity, stating that parasites are more active around the time of the full moon each month. I never gave much validity to this theory as I have felt parasitic activity within my body at all times during the month, not just near the full moon phase. Whether the parasites are more active around the full moon still remains speculation. However, I did conduct an experiment with this theory, paying much closer attention to what I was feeling within my body during all times of the month and during the full moon. I researched to find out that the next full moon was going to be on January 23rd, and I did pass a very large parasite before then on January 18th. Although, I felt anal itching much of the entire month and was passing some parasites, I felt the most uncomfortable anal itching and worms crawling inside of my anus more so around the days of the full moon or new moon. On the actual day of the full moon, I felt anal itching all day long, not just at night. I do not have scientific proof that this is a valid theory, I am just telling you what I felt based upon my own experimentation with the parasite cleanse during the month. Pay attention to your own body and what you are feeling during various days, keep a journal if necessary.

Because of the full moon theory increasing parasitic activity, it wouldn't hurt to continue the parasite cleanse throughout a full 6-week time frame that spans across a full moon cycle just in case this theory is valid. It is said that parasites lay more eggs and become more active just before and after the full moon, so continuing your cleanse through this time period should help to eradicate the parasites.

The parasite cleanse should be continued for 6 weeks and then take a break before starting again. I had been doing the parasite cleanses off and on for years, but when I finally combined ingredients is when I experienced the greatest results with expelling parasites. Here are a few pictures of a parasite that I expelled in January of 2016. If you take a close look at the pictures below, it appears that there may be a few wrapped together in a rope formation. Although, after passing this parasite, I still felt a lot of anal itching so I know that there were more inside of me.

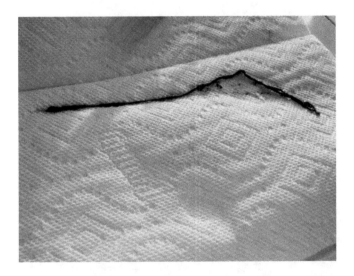

Figure 6: Parasite expelled January 2016

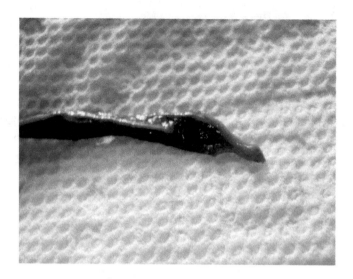

Figure 7: closer picture of parasite

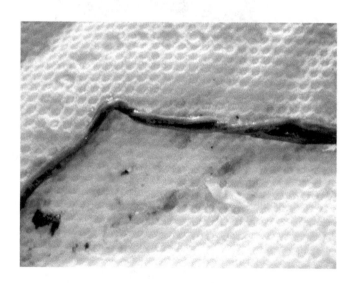

Figure 8: different view of parasite

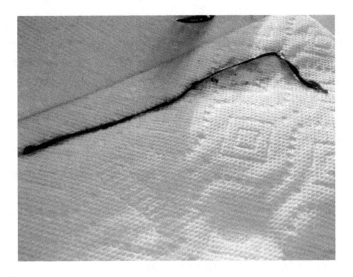

Figure 9: different view of parasite

Ingredients needed for the Parasite Cleanse:

Digestive Enzymes: Protease is a digestive enzyme which digests protein. The reason for using this enzyme is too digest parasites as parasites are made up of protein. The higher the HUT value in the protease, the more effective it will work toward gobbling up the protein that are parasites. I take digestive enzymes with a high protease HUT value before each meal and also at night before bed.

The brand I currently use is Doctor's Best Digestive Enzymes with a protease level of 95,000 HUT per 1 capsule. I take 2 capsules before breakfast, 2 before lunch, 2 before dinner and then I also take 2 before bedtime. That is a total of 760,000 HUT of protease per day. Sometimes I vary this number and take more digestive enzymes before each meal.

Cloves: Clove will kill the eggs of the parasites only, so this needs to be used in conjunction with wormwood and black walnut in order for it to be effective at killing parasites. I usually take 1 clove capsule in the morning, 1 before lunch, 1 before dinner and 1 at bedtime. I have varied this dosage at times to be 2, 2, 2, and 2.

95

Cloves can aid in digestion, soothe the inner lining of the intestines, act as an expectorant, relieves tooth pain, kills parasites and bacteria in the digestive tract, relieve excess gas and bloating, can be used as an antihistamine, relieves pain from rheumatism, arthritis and inflammatory pain. (21).

Wormwood: Wormwood kills the adults and developmental stages of the parasites, so it is important to use this in conjunction with clove and black walnut to make sure to kill the parasites and the eggs.

I usually take 2 wormwood capsules before breakfast, 2 before lunch, 2 before dinner and then 2 at bedtime. There are also wormwood combination capsules which combine the wormwood, black walnut and cloves.

Wormwood is "useful in alleviating fever, expelling parasitic worms like roundworm from the digestive tract, and for its tonic effects. It may also be applied topically to reduce inflammation of insect bites and promote healing. Wormwood is also noted to be useful in treating jaundice, a sign of liver dysfunction and to increase sexual desire." (22).

Black Walnut: The Black Walnut offers many medicinal uses and benefits; it is anti-parasitic, anti-bacterial, anti-fungal and anti-viral. It can also be used for parasites, candida, eczema, psoriasis, jock itch, athlete's foot, ringworm, herpes, warts, cold sores, sore throat, and is also an anti-cancer compound. (23).

Black Walnut also kills the adults and developmental stages of the parasite, so it must be used in conjunction with clove and wormwood to make sure to kill the parasites and the eggs.

I usually take 2 black walnut capsules before breakfast, 2 before lunch, 2 before dinner and then 2 at bedtime. There are also wormwood combination capsules which combine the wormwood, black walnut and cloves.

Neem Leaf: Neem is a tree; native of India, which consists of the root, bark, leaves, seed, fruit, and flower. Neem is known to kill parasites, viruses, bacterial and fungal infections. Neem is also an anti-fertility herb and is used as a birth control method, which may cause abortions and infertility. DO NOT take Neem if you are pregnant, breast feeding, or trying to get pregnant.

"The Neem leaf is used for leprosy, stomach upset, eye disorders, diabetes, fever, gum disease, liver problems, birth control, abortions, and intestinal worms. The Neem bark is used for malaria, stomach ulcers, intestinal ulcers, skin diseases, pain, and ulcers. The Neem flower is used for intestinal worms, controlling phlegm and reducing bile flow. The Fruit of the Neem tree is used for hemorrhoids, urinary tract disorders, intestinal worms, diabetes, wounds, bloody nose, phlegm, eye disorders and leprosy. The twigs of the Neem tree are used by the natives to brush their teeth as they chew on the twig. The twig is also beneficial for intestinal worms, cough, asthma, hemorrhoids, urinary disorders, and diabetes." (12). Neem oil is used for leprosy, abortions, birth control, psoriasis, eczema and intestinal worms.

Neem can help to kill parasites in the intestinal tract. (12). Neem is also an excellent insect repellant and it doesn't contain harsh chemicals. I personally use Neem face cream daily and use Neem lotion on exposed skin when going out for a hike in the woods to naturally repel the bugs and ticks. Using Neem can help to keep mosquitoes and other insects at bay and is a great natural insect repellant without using harsh chemicals on the skin.

More benefits of Neem include lowering blood sugar levels, which can help those with diabetes. Those with diabetes should monitor their blood sugar carefully when using Neem. Children should not use Neem Oil by mouth due to serious side effects "include vomiting, diarrhea, drowsiness, blood disorders, seizures, loss of consciousness, coma, brain disorders, and death." (12).

Sometimes, I take the dosage of black walnut, wormwood, cloves, Neem, diatomaceous earth and protease (digestive) enzymes. Then I switch it up with dosage on all of those, sometimes varying between only taking Neem one day, then something else another day, sometimes I skip a day to let the parasites think that they are safe, then go the next day with a higher dosage to kill those who became active overnight.

According to WebMD; You should not take Neem internally for longer than 10 weeks.

During the parasite cleanse; I take 2 Neem capsules before breakfast, 2 before lunch, 2 before dinner and 2 at bedtime. Sometimes I vary this by only taking 1 capsule of Neem at breakfast, lunch, dinner and bedtime.

Diatomaceous Earth: Diatomaceous Earth is another way to eradicate parasites from the body and it is also safe for pets. You want to make sure that you only use food grade diatomaceous earth, not the pool grade. The food grade

will say that it is safe for pets on the label. You should treat your cat or dog for parasites at the same time that you are detoxifying yourself from parasites, so you won't re-infest yourself or your animals. (13).

Diatomaceous earth is made from the skeletal remains of hard shelled algae known as diatoms. (14). The mineral composition of diatomaceous earth is 80% silica, 10% metal oxides (magnesium, aluminum, calcium) and 10% moisture. The food grade diatomaceous earth is purified by washing it and removing the metal oxides leaving behind primarily silica. (14). The mineral is ground into fine, tiny fragments and shards which cut the insects/parasites once they run across it. (13). You must not breathe in the diatomaceous earth as it can harm the tiny villi in the lung.

Another use for diatomaceous earth is as an insect repellant. It is good to use for ants or other bugs inside the house and it is non-toxic to animals or humans. You can sprinkle the diatomaceous earth around the perimeter of your home to keep out any bugs because when the bugs walk across the line of diatomaceous earth, they get cut up and die.

Aside from the diatomaceous earth killing parasites within the body, a great benefit I have found is that it makes the hair and nails grow really fast due to the high silica content. My nails get really long and strong when I am taking diatomaceous earth. There was also a time when I was losing huge chunks of hair in the shower daily due to a low thyroid and hormonal imbalance, taking diatomaceous earth daily helped to stop my hair from falling out and my hair started re-growing healthy and thick again.

I would take 1 Tablespoon of diatomaceous earth in 8 ounces of water and drink immediately before the diatomaceous earth settles to the bottom. Take this mixture two to three times per day to get rid of parasites, usually once in the morning and once before bedtime. You can take 1 Tablespoon in water per day for a maintenance dose after the parasites are gone. The diatomaceous earth will help to rid the digestive tract and colon of the parasites.

In regards to detoxifying your pets from fleas and parasites, make sure to give your cat or dog ½ to 1 teaspoon of Diatomaceous earth once per day for 90 days, depending upon the weight of your pet. As mentioned previously, it is a good idea to detoxify both yourself and your pets at the same time so you won't get re-infested with parasites. Also make sure to wash all bedding, carpeting, and sprinkle diatomaceous earth around bedding or carpeting or in the litter box, wherever the parasites may have dropped.

According to Wolf Creek Ranch Animal Sanctuary, they use diatomaceous earth daily to rid their animals of worms and they don't skip a day because if you skip a few days of feeding diatomaceous earth, the dead and dying worms emit bacteria, toxins and ammonia which can make pets and people sicker due to the die off. (13). This is why it is important to continue diatomaceous earth for at least 90 days. I personally use the Good Pet brand of food grade diatomaceous earth and have given it to my cats. Follow all instructions on the label when using diatomaceous earth. Make sure to always use food grade, as diatomaceous earth also has a pool grade that is mixed with chemicals and is not fit for human or animal consumption.

There are also parasite cleanse kits on the market which may be easier to do if you are new to detoxing. The parasite kits work the same as a colon cleanse kit or a candida cleanse kit, where you take pills or powders from a package specified by the directions on the box. Make sure that the parasite cleansing kit at least contains the ingredients of clove, wormwood, and black walnut to ensure effective cleansing of the adult parasites, larvae, and eggs.

Pumpkin Seeds (Pepitas): Pumpkin seeds; also known as Pepitas must be eaten raw for it to be effective. Pumpkin seeds may not actually kill off the parasite but the pumpkin seed contains "high levels of compounds known as cucurbitins, which paralyze the worms. This prevents them from holding on to the intestinal walls, as they usually do during a bowel movement." (7).

"Pumpkin seed is a beta-carotene-rich supplement and high in antioxidant vitamins A, C and E, many valuable minerals (especially zinc), amino acids (including the rare amino acid called myosin and the unusual cucurbitin, which is very helpful for worm infestations), essential fatty acids and dietary fiber." (15).

Beneficial Uses of Pumpkin Seeds:

Another way to cleanse parasites from your intestinal tract is too use raw pumpkin seeds; otherwise known as pepitas, which are known for expelling worms. (5). Raw pumpkin seeds will be green in color, make sure to get them raw and not roasted. "Pumpkin Seeds are known to be an effective and powerful anthelmintic that will kill and expel worm infestations in children and adults. The unusual amino acid; cucurbitin, in pumpkin seeds are said to make the herb one of the most efficient remedies for killing intestinal parasites, including tapeworms and roundworms." (15).

I grind up ½ cup (specifically during a parasite cleanse) of pumpkin seeds in a vitamix or coffee grinder and add them to a morning smoothie or you can grind up ½ cup and add it to oatmeal. Another idea is to add it too yogurt to make it more palatable. You can also put the fine pumpkin grind into a bowl and add coconut milk until it becomes thick like oatmeal consistency. You can eat this and drink plenty of water afterward. Do this in the morning on an empty stomach. You then take the liquid bentonite clay or the Triphala capsules or powder at night before bed.

The pumpkin seeds will help to dislodge the worms from the intestinal tract and the liquid bentonite clay or Triphala will help to expel them from your body. I have personally experimented with this, also adding the pumpkin seed mixture to a morning smoothie so I can drink it easier. When you are in between parasite cleanses, you can use 1-2 Tablespoons of ground pumpkin seeds in a smoothie to keep parasites away and boost your zinc levels.

Humaworm Experiment: Even after repeating the parasite cleanse for over six weeks and expelling parasites, I could still feel parasites inside of me, so I switched up the treatment again and experimented with Humaworm for 30 days. Here are the results: I also got a large worm out while using Humaworm the first time for 30 days. Follow the instructions on the package for Humaworm. Although, instead of waiting only ½ hour to eat, I would wait at least an hour to give more time for the Humaworm to work at killing the parasites. After completing Humaworm for 30 days, I took a 30-day break but still felt some parasitic activity. I repeated Humaworm once again for 30 days but the parasites do become accustomed to various herbal cleanses, so it is imperative to keep switching up the parasite cleansing routine. If you are heavily infested with parasites, you will need to continue parasite cleansing for up to a year, with taking 30 day breaks in between various cleanses.

After completing my parasite cleanse above, then 2 rounds of Humaworm, my parasitic activity was still present but too a much lesser degree, although I still was getting negative testing results on stool samples. I repeated another round of parasite cleanses and finally the itching had gone away and I felt no more parasitic activity. Although, just to be sure, I did wait an extra 30 days and then resumed one more parasite cleanse for 30 days just in case eggs had hatched during that time.

Although you can do the over the counter parasite cleansing kit, it is not safe for animals as is food grade diatomaceous earth. So, if you choose the over the counter kit for yourself, give your animals the food grade diatomaceous earth at the same time. Depending upon the level of parasitic infestation in your pets, you may need to use the over-the-counter worm medicine for your pet or take your pet to the veterinarian for a set of liquid or pills that eradicate the parasites.

If you do not eradicate the parasites in your pets, they will keep spreading the worms to you and vice versa. I am almost certain that I got parasites from my cats as I always rescue cats from the shelters and usually they are infested with worms. I adopted my last cat at the end of 2014 and he was so heavily infested with worms that nothing worked on him until I finally had to take him to the veterinarian to have multiple treatments for parasites. I had kept up the parasite cleanses on and off throughout the past couple of years but with severe leaky gut, it is difficult to eradicate the parasites until after the gut lining is healed.

Another great way to eradicate parasites is the parasite enema, which helps for those who feel the worms crawling and moving around near the anus at night where it keeps you awake. I had this happen to me and the parasites would wake me up around 1:00 am and keep me up all night. I could actually feel the worms crawling around inside of my anus. I got so irritated by the worms keeping me awake that I did a parasite enema which calmed them down and most likely killed them quickly. Make sure that when you feel these worms crawling around your anus that you DO NOT itch anywhere around the anus because then you could easily get parasite parts and eggs underneath your nails, your clothing or bedding and spread parasites elsewhere.

Below is a list of various enemas which can also help to eradicate parasitic activity within the colon.

Parasite Enema #1:

I add the ingredients directly to a coffee enema (see the liver detox chapter for the coffee enema mixture).

- 10 drops of clove oil
- 10 drops of wormwood
- 10 drops of black walnut hull

All of this is mixed into the coffee in the enema bag. Hold the mixture for at least 15 minutes before releasing into the toilet, this is a retention enema.

Parasite Enema #2:

I add the ingredients directly to a coffee enema (see the liver detox chapter for the coffee enema mixture).

- 2 Tablespoons of Plantation brand unsulphured blackstrap molasses
- 10-20 drops of garlic oil (you can either mash garlic cloves and pour in the juice or they sell garlic oil, which I find much easier because mashed garlic gets stuck in the enema tube)

All of this is mixed into the coffee in the enema bag. Hold the mixture for at least 15 minutes, this is a retention enema. Sometimes I will also mix some Neem Oil into the enema bag. Either of these enemas works great to stop the itching immediately so you can get some sleep.

You can and should do the parasite cleanse and the candida cleanse at the same time unless you have chronic candida and are heavily infested with parasites, then you may need to do them separately so you won't release too many toxins into the body at one time. Make sure to support your liver during the process by increasing the liver cleansing foods, liver supplement or even lemon water daily.

Below is a story from a friend of mine who was suffering with parasitic infection for years. This picture below is of a two-and-a-half-foot dead rope worm, which came out of a friend of mine during a colon hydrotherapy session, the hydrotherapist took a picture of this nasty creature which was living inside of her causing her all types of health issues, below is her story. You could have these parasites living inside of you right now and not even know it; this is why it is so important to do a regular detox for parasites.

Jane's Story:

Jane Doe (name changed for anonymity) had begun having blisters on the palms of her hands back in 2000. Her palms became raw to the point of bleeding. She had been to see countless doctors and not one could tell her what the problem was, the doctors just kept giving her prescription creams, all of which never worked. Finally, she went to a Naturopathic doctor who suggested that the peeling palms that bled had to do with parasitic infection and that she should look into hydrotherapy to fix her issue. That is where she began to look into detoxification to heal her parasite condition.

Other symptoms that Jane had experienced in the latter years where she was always constipated, and her stomach was bloated, hard, and gassy. When Jane would lie on her back, her stomach would expand and contract in the intestinal area. She could actually feel and see the parasite moving within her stomach/intestinal area. That is when the parasite was active within her intestines.

Jane reluctantly began going to a colon hydrotherapist to hopefully fix her parasite problem. The colonics were getting rid of smaller worms within her system, but she still had issues within her body and knew that she had a larger parasite causing her issues. Jane had continued with the hydrotherapist for three years, who put her on specific enzymes to kill the parasites. After three full years, Jane had finally experienced a massive pain in her chest for 3 days straight. She knew that it wasn't a heart issue but a die off reaction of the worm dying off within her system. After the 3 days of pain, Jane went for another colon hydrotherapy session and finally one of the rope worms released from her colon and came out. The picture below is of the actual rope worm in the colon hydrotherapist tube immediately after releasing from Jane's body.

The rope worm has suction cups which attach to the intestinal walls and feed off the hosts' nutrient supply. Jane had continuously done parasite cleanses which had eventually weakened the rope worm over the years to finally release. Jane had two large rope worms released, the first one in August of 2012 and the second large rope worm released in February of 2014. To have rope worms this large, they had obviously been growing in her system for many years, as she had symptoms back in 2000. Other symptoms Jane experienced were food cravings of salt. She also had a large blister on the arch of her right food, which both cleared up at the passing of the ropeworms.

Jane stuck to a strict diet of no gluten, no sugar, and no dairy while she was cleansing her body of parasites. She eats mainly a vegan/vegetarian diet and mostly raw vegetables. She would also juice 32 ounces of green juice daily, rotating her greens, with beets, and wheatgrass. However, this experience had left her very fearful of eating at times because of the fear of another parasitic invasion. Her boyfriend, who is a doctor, also had to do parasite cleansing because they can re-infect one another.

After the rope worms released from Jane's colon, her hands cleared up, the skin cleared up, her hair started growing back healthier and she now has more energy. Jane continues on her path to wellness using only alternative methods by enlisting in periodic detoxing and detoxing for parasites. She also continues her vegan/vegetarian diet eating mostly raw foods.

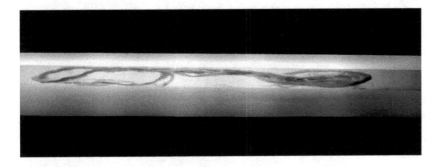

Figure 10: Rope worm inside of colon hydrotherapist tube

How long should I continue the parasite cleanse?

This is dependent upon your personal health issues. I have personally continued the parasite cleanse off and on for the past eight years and will continue to do so until I feel the parasites are gone completely. Since test results aren't very reliable and the testing is $400 dollars each time, makes it financially not feasible for many people to test daily for months to get a positive parasite test. When you do a parasite cleanse, stick with it for at least 6 weeks so you cover the time frame where parasites may be more active at certain times of the month. Although the theory is that parasites are more active during full moon phases,

I have felt them and expelled them at other times during the lunar cycle, but just in case this theory is true, six weeks of continual parasite cleansing wouldn't hurt.

You may need to repeat the parasite cleanse multiple times throughout the year, for years, until your symptoms clear up. The main thing is too listen to your body and pay attention to the signs and symptoms. Keep a journal of which symptoms you have, what you eat, and the cleanse you are doing to see if there are any positive or negative changes. Keeping a journal is the easiest way to begin to learn how to read your body properly.

After you have successfully completed the colon, candida, and parasite cleanses, you can move onto the kidney cleanse. Keep in mind that you may need to repeat the candida cleanse and the parasite cleanse for quite a while before you move onto the kidney cleanse. Another option is to complete the entire order of individual cleanses first, and then go back to repeat the ones which may still be burdening you (for many that may be candida and parasites).

9

The Kidney Cleanse

The two kidneys lie in the back of the abdominal wall and play a central role in regulating the body's water, salt, potassium, and acid concentration within the body. (1). The kidneys also remove metabolic waste from the blood excreting it into the urine. (1).

The kidney cleanse will help to rid the kidneys of kidney stones and will help the kidneys to work efficiently. In order to cleanse the kidneys, you can brew a tea made of parsley. Put 4 bunches of fresh parsley into a quart of water and bring to a boil. Let the mixture cool a bit and drink ½ cup of parsley tea daily for 3 weeks.

There are also pre-made teas on the market that are specifically designed for a kidney detox, which contain parsley and/or uva ursi and can also be used to aid in detoxifying the kidneys. You can also find kidney detox kits in a health food store. The common herbs and foods used to detoxify the kidneys are; Dandelion, Marshmallow root, Juniper, Nettles, Parsley, Red Clover, Ginger, Uva Ursi, Goldenrod, Watermelon, Lemon Juice, Cranberry Juice, Beet Juice, and Pumpkin Seeds. (2). If you are using cranberry juice in conjunction with a kidney cleanse, make sure that your cranberry juice is free from sugar or high fructose corn syrup.

Another way to cleanse the kidneys is to add parsley and/or dandelion greens to your juicing regimen. Cranberry Juice or Beet Juice also helps to cleanse the kidneys. Lemon juice can also help to stop oxalate crystals from forming in the kidneys, which is the cause of kidney stones. So, by adding some lemon juice to your water daily you are helping to combat kidney stones. In the case that you do get kidney stones, here is a great natural remedy to get rid of them quickly.

Kidney Stones Natural Remedy:

If you want to get rid of kidney stones, you can use 1 cup of olive oil mixed with 1 cup of freshly squeezed lemon juice. This combination will help the kidney stones to pass on their own.

I had kidney stones back in November of 2013 and was just about ready to drive myself to the emergency room when I found this healing gem. For a few consecutive days, I felt immense pain around my kidneys. At first, I thought it was just lower back pain, but it didn't go away and continued to get so bad that I could barely walk and was in tears. I finally figured that I may have a kidney stone, so I took this olive oil/lemon juice combination a few times within a 24-hour period and passed the kidney stones and a gallstone the next day. The pain stopped immediately after passing the stones. If you have kidney stones, you may feel nauseous when taking this recipe, but it will pass. Below is a picture of kidney stones.

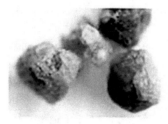

Figure 11: kidney stones magnified

I have also found a wonderful supplement which helps keep kidney and gallbladder stones away for good. The kidney supplement is called "Stone Free" from Planetary Herbals. This supplement is a great addition to add to your daily regimen during and after completing a kidney cleanse because it increases bile flow, which is also beneficial for the liver. After completing the Kidney Cleanse, you can move on to the Liver cleanse, which is the last organ that should be cleansed.

10

The Liver Cleanse

Now that you have completed all of the other cleanses, you have cleared the channels of elimination to make way for the liver cleanse. The liver cleanse should be the last organ on your list of cleanses. Many people suffer from allergies, asthma, cystic acne, fibromyalgia, cancer, chronic migraines and a host of other conditions. The reasons for these conditions are not only stemming from candida overgrowth but can also be related to an overabundance of gallstones which are clogging your liver. Even if you had your gallbladder removed, it is still possible to have gallstones clogging the liver. These stones that clog your liver can cause health problems and most all cancer patients have a clogged liver, so it is important to detoxify this organ.

The Liver is one of the largest organs of the body which can convert nutrients in our diets into substances our bodies can use and it also takes toxic substances in our bodies and converts them into harmless substances or makes sure those toxins are released from the body. (1). The problems arise when we become chronically ill with cancer or other diseases that may release a large amount of toxic material that the liver can become overburdened with toxins all trying to be released at once. Some of the toxins will be released from the body by the liver but when the liver is overburdened with toxins, some of those toxins can be re-released back into the body causing more damage and chronic illness. If the toxins do not get released from the liver, it can cause extreme inflammation, liver damage and even death. This is one of the reasons that you will often see many people who are being treated with chemotherapy (a carcinogen), bloat up like a balloon due to the mass amounts of toxins trying to be released at once and the liver cannot handle all of the toxins at once so those toxins get re-circulated back into the body causing the extreme inflammation and many times death.

You may also have gallstones clogging your liver if you have ever taken prescription medication, birth control pills, drank excessive amounts of alcohol, hepatitis, cirrhosis, taken illegal drugs, chemotherapy, radiation, or have or have had cancer. This liver cleanse was designed by Dr. Hulda Clark, with a few additions to maximize the benefits, and works great but can be exhausting. Make sure that you have nothing to do the evening and day after the liver cleanse, as you will be rather tired from performing this cleanse. Although, the benefit of this cleanse is that it only lasts one day and then you can go on with your life, so it is easy to do when you have a couple of days off from work. It is very important that you do not jump to this cleanse, you MUST do the other cleanses in proper order or the channels of elimination may not be clear to do this cleanse successfully.

How to do the Liver Cleanse:

Do not eat anything after 2:00 pm the day you begin the liver cleanse. You will need Epsom Salt, Olive Oil, Organic Pink Grapefruit juice, Black Walnut tincture, Ornithine Capsules, and liquid Bentonite clay. You may also want to have extra towels to lie on while you are sleeping in case of an accident in the middle of the night. Here is a timeline of how to successfully perform a liver cleanse.

2:00 pm: mix together 3 cups of purified water and 4 Tablespoons of Epsom Salt in a large container. Put the mixture in the refrigerator to chill for the 6:00 pm start. 2:00 pm is also the time you will stop eating for the day.

6:00 pm: Drink ¾ cup of the Epsom Salt mixture.

8:00 pm: Drink ¾ cup of the Epsom Salt mixture.

9:45 pm: Mix ½ cup of Olive Oil with ½ cup of Organic Pink grapefruit juice and 20 drops of Black Walnut tincture into a glass jar, close the jar and shake the mixture. Take 8 Ornithine capsules with a glass of water. You can also take a melatonin or 5 HTP to help you sleep if you don't think the Ornithine capsules will be enough. Visit the bathroom once more.

10:00 pm: Shake the oil/grapefruit mixture again until watery and drink with a straw within 5 minutes, then immediately go lay down on your right side with your right knee up to your chest. This will help the gallstones flow down the biliary duct. Sleep until 6:00 am laying on your right side. It is a good idea to lay some old towels down on your bed in case of an accident during the night.

6:00 am: Drink ¾ cup of the Epsom Salt mixture. You may go back to bed. Make sure to lay on your right side and lay the towels down under your buttocks in case of an accident.

8:00 am: Drink the last ¾ cup of the Epsom Salt mixture. This is when I find the most activity begins to happen between 8:00 am and 10:00 am when you may be running to the bathroom passing gallstones, although everyone's experience may be different.

10:00 am: You may now eat something but try to make it light. I usually eat some fruit and maybe some scrambled eggs or gluten free oatmeal.

When you visit the bathroom in the morning, you may see gallstones floating to the top of the toilet. The gallstones will vary in color and size depending upon your level of toxicity. The gallstones can be dark green, light green, bright green, or yellow in color. If you have passed any gallstones, you will need to repeat this liver cleanse every few months until all of the gallstones have been eliminated.

A hint while doing this cleanse, when you start passing gallstones or right before, take a few ounces of Liquid Bentonite Clay with a large glass of lukewarm water. This will help to soak up any toxins that may get re-released back into your body. When the gallstones start releasing from the liver, toxins can be re-released back into the body and you want to avoid this so as not to cause further problems. This is a very important step and should not be skipped.

You didn't accumulate these gallstones overnight, so this process may take quite a few repeats to eliminate all of the gallstones clogging your liver. When I had cancer, I had passed over 1,800 stones and it took almost 6 months of cleanses to do it, passing approximately 150-200 stones per cleanse. I had also conducted this cleanse in 2017, when I no longer had cancer, and only ended up passing about 25-30 stones. The Liver Cleanse will help you to eliminate allergies, asthma, have clearer skin, and eliminate other ailments for good.

I had made a mistake while doing this cleanse when I had cancer, as I was repeating this liver cleanse every two weeks, instead of once every few months, and not taking the Bentonite clay to absorb the toxins. What had happened is that I had re-released too many toxins back into my body and created other health problems; such as severe intestinal permeability (leaky gut syndrome), Irritable Bowel Syndrome (IBS), asthma, high cortisol, hormonal imbalance, low thyroid, extreme weight gain, and eventually my adrenal glands crashed causing advanced adrenal fatigue due to lowered immune function creating too much stress upon my body. This is why it is important to only do this cleanse every few months and utilize the liquid Bentonite clay as a buffer to aid in soaking up excess toxins.

In addition to adding the liquid Bentonite clay to this liver cleanse, it is a good idea to follow up with coffee enemas to flush out the additional gallstones, which didn't leave the body during the cleanse. I personally like to do 3 coffee enemas the day of the liver flush, after you have passed the gallstones after 10:00 am. And then follow up with 2 coffee enemas per day until you notice less gallstones floating in the toilet.

Another way to detoxify the liver is to take extra doses of milk thistle capsules, 600 mg of Alpha Lipoic Acid, Niacin, turmeric powder or capsules, Uva Ursi, beets, beet greens, NAC, stone free from planetary herbals, and dandelion greens. You can add these to your daily juicing regimen or take them on their own. You can also find liver detox teas (Yogi makes a dandelion tea and so does Teecino), liver tonics, and liver detoxification kits either online or at your local health food store. All will help to detoxify the liver in a more gradual manner. For those with chronic conditions, you will need more than just milk thistle or turmeric to rid the liver of all of the toxins burdening the system. This is where the liver cleanses and the coffee enema comes into play.

Coffee Enema Liver Detox:

The coffee enema will sound crazy to most people, as it did to me at first, until you learn about the history and benefits. I swore up and down that I would never do a coffee enema and then I broke down and did one and can't imagine a detoxification regimen without it, especially if you are trying to heal from cancer or other chronic conditions in where your liver may become overburdened with toxins.

The benefits of coffee enemas were accidentally discovered in World War I, when a nurse in the hospital accidentally filled a soldier's enema bag with coffee instead of water. According to Dr. Lawrence Wilson, who quoted an article written by Gar Hildenbrand, in the Healing Newsletter in 1986, the story goes like this:

"The coffee enema may have been first used in modern Western nations as a pain reliever. As the story goes, during World War I nurses kept coffee pots on the stove all day long. The battle surgeons and others drank it to stay awake while working horrendously long hours. Enema bags hung around as some patients needed help moving their bowels. There was a severe shortage of pain medications. So, they were forced to save the pain drugs for surgical procedures with little or none for follow-up after surgery. When surgical patients woke up from operations without the benefit of further morphine injections they would scream in pain and agony from the surgery, and they would be constipated as well from the anesthesia drugs. For the constipation, a nurse was preparing an enema for constipation. Instead of fetching water for the enema, she accidentally dumped some cool coffee into the patient's enema bag, released the clamp, and into the patient it flowed. "I'm not in so much pain," the poor soldier said. It was a coffee enema moment in history. Thus began the use of coffee enemas to help control pain." (5).

Since there was a shortage of pain medication in World War I, the hospital began using coffee enemas. Coffee enemas were even utilized for pain and written in the Merck manual, used by doctors, until the 1970's when the coffee enema and its benefits were taken out of the Merck manual. My theory is western allopathic medicine figured out that the coffee enema was detoxifying the liver and healing patients of cancer, pain, and other diseases to which their toxic drugs were no longer needed.

Dr. Max Gerson, who created the Gerson therapy for Cancer and other diseases, utilized coffee enemas to detoxify the liver and manage pain, for advanced cancer patients, along with fresh vegetable juices to heal the body naturally. The coffee enema works to increase the bile flow from the liver, thus increasing glutathione and detoxifying the liver of harmful toxins. This liver detox is easy to do and is very relaxing once you get the hang of it.

You will need an enema bag; I bought mine at Wal-Mart for around $5.00. You must only use organic coffee because it contains no chemicals, which are utilized during the processing of regular coffee. The organic coffee is very important because your colon will soak up whatever you put into it and you do not want chemicals from regular coffee soaking into your body. Your goal is to get the toxins out, not put them back in.

To start the coffee enema, you will brew a pot of organic coffee with purified water (not tap water) and then let the coffee cool. I used to make the coffee at night before bed and then use it first thing in the morning after the coffee had cooled overnight. To do a coffee enema, fill the enema bag with the brewed room temperature, organic coffee and hang the filled bag a couple of feet above the bathroom floor. Lay a large towel down in the bathroom and get comfortable with a timer and something to read. Make sure to lie on your right-hand side, as this is the side where your liver is located. Use a little coconut oil or lubricant on the end of the insertion tip. Insert the tip and gently let a cup or two of coffee run into the colon. Stop the flow of coffee, from the clasp on the enema bag, if you feel too much pressure. During the enema, while you are holding the coffee, if you feel pressure like you are going to have a bowel movement, breathe deeply until the pressure subsides. You will

114

find over time, how much coffee is comfortable for you to hold without getting pressure. Some people can hold more coffee and some less, this will take practice until you find what is comfortable for you.

It is a wise decision to do a quick enema first to get any fecal matter out of the colon first, which will make it easier to be able to hold the coffee enema for the full 15-20 minutes. The coffee enema should be held for at least 15-20 minutes, so the gallbladder will release toxins into the liver and the liver will then release its toxins by increasing bile flow. If you begin to cramp, you can take deep breaths and the cramp will usually subside.

You can also massage the entire length of the colon and small intestines while performing the coffee enema. This will help to release any dried or old fecal matter that may be stuck within the pockets in the colon. This can also help to release any parasitic nests that may be in your small intestines as well. Don't feel bad if you can't hold the coffee enema the entire 20 minutes, this takes practice. Through experimentation, I have noticed that I can hold more coffee when I have done a quick enema first, do the enema after I have a bowel movement or when I haven't ingested enough water throughout the day and am dehydrated. Because your colon soaks up what you put into it, if you are dehydrated, it will soak up the water from the coffee. This is why it is imperative to use only filtered or bottled water when brewing the organic coffee.

The more you perform this cleanse, the easier it will become. In time, you will be able to feel and hear a noise of the gallbladder releasing into the liver, which sounds like a gurgle or burping noise. The coffee enema can be done a few times a day but make sure that you are drinking vegetable broths or fresh vegetable juices after the enemas to replace any minerals lost. You can also eat a banana or avocado to replace the potassium levels lost during the coffee enema.

I have discovered that the coffee enema also works very well when you are detoxifying the body because it helps to flush the liver of toxins. For instance, whenever I have decided to stop drinking coffee, I would go through caffeine withdrawals which would lead to a monster sized migraine headache. Doing a coffee enema shortens the length of time that you experience withdrawals and gets rid of the headache very quickly by releasing toxins from the liver. This trick also works if you are out for a night of partying; ingesting too many alcoholic beverages and you don't want a hangover the next day. The reason people get a hangover is because their liver is overburdened with the toxic effects of the alcohol, so using the coffee enema to flush the toxins just makes sense.

The withdrawals you experience from detoxing the body are due to the liver being overburdened with toxins, which the liver is trying to cart out of the body. By doing the coffee enema, you are just helping the body to flush the liver of those toxins. If you leave the toxins in the liver and your liver becomes overburdened with toxins, it can re-intoxicate your system and cause inflammation and further health problems. This is why a coffee enema is vital for those with cancer or other chronic diseases where there will be many toxins being processed through the liver during a detoxification process.

Before I started doing coffee enemas I had already went through Cancer twice and was on my death bed. This is the main reason why I experienced extreme inflammation after the second bout with cancer as my liver was overburdened and those toxins had nowhere to go except for back into my body and my cells, creating extreme inflammation and many other chronic conditions which I was left to heal naturally.

As you can see, there are quite a number of various liver cleanses. Start slowly with the liver cleanses as if you do a liver cleanse too fast it will release too many toxins back into the system which may cause other health issues to deal with. Try the different types of liver cleanses to see which one works best for you.

Glutathione & the Liver:

I have already discussed a bit about glutathione and the liver in regard to the benefits of coffee enemas, but what exactly is glutathione and how does it detoxify your liver?

Glutathione is the master detoxifier of the liver and gallbladder. You cannot get glutathione from a pill or a patch, but your body has to produce it from the foods you eat.

Although there are many companies out there that will try to sell you a glutathione pill or a patch, they are a waste of money, in my opinion. I discussed in the previous section the benefits of the coffee enema and how it increases glutathione production to the liver, which aids to detoxify the liver.

Another great way to increase glutathione production within your body is through turmeric, milk thistle, whey protein powder, and dandelion. You can also increase glutathione production through the amino acid L-glutamine, which also helps to heal intestinal permeability (aka; leaky gut syndrome). The various foods that help to increase glutathione production within the body are avocado, whey protein, eggs, l-glutamine, turmeric, milk thistle, and dandelion.

I usually take turmeric by the teaspoon, mixed into a glass of lukewarm water and drunken down quickly, followed by a bit of water to wash the taste of the turmeric out of my mouth. I found I save a lot of money by buying my turmeric in bulk from an Indian or Middle Eastern grocery store, as opposed to buying turmeric supplements. Through my experimentation, I noticed that ingesting turmeric, to increase glutathione production, helps to break up gallstones naturally, aids in repairing intestinal permeability, heals boils & cystic acne, and heals irritable bowel syndrome (IBS) quickly.

Foods and Herbs that Detoxify the Liver:

In conjunction with doing a liver cleanse, it is a good idea to add these liver cleansing foods to your daily diet throughout all of the individual detoxes in order to support the liver. These liver cleansing foods can help to increase the glutathione; the master detoxifier, within the body. The following foods, herbs, and supplements are known to help cleanse the liver; beets, turmeric, milk thistle, alpha lipoic acid, niacin, N-acetyl cysteine (NAC), burdock root, dandelion, garlic, grapefruit, carrots, arugula, mustard greens, chicory root, cranberries, spinach, avocados, broccoli, lemons, limes, cauliflower, olive oil, apples, apple cider vinegar (with the mother), and cabbage.

While conducting the other detoxes or even if you are healing leaky gut, adrenal fatigue, SIBO or other infections, it is a good idea to support the liver detox pathways even with squeezing fresh lemon juice into your water daily and adding some Bragg's apple cider vinegar to your daily regime.

Probiotic Retention Enema:

This enema will help to restore functionality to the colon, heal the intestinal lining and restore good bacteria within the colon.

Ingredients:

- 1 tsp Natren's Digesta Lac Powder
- 1 tsp Natren's Bifidofactor Powder
- 1 tsp Natren's Megadopholous Powder
- 1 cup Lily of the Desert or George's Aloe Vera Juice Stomach formula
- ½ cup of Cold Pressed Flax Seed Oil

Add all ingredients into a bowl and mix with a wire whisk. Pour the mixture into a clean enema bag. Make sure to perform a cleansing enema; to clear the colon of fecal matter prior to using the retention enema. Put a bit of coconut oil on your rectum or on the tip of the enema tube or both, whichever is most comfortable for you? Lay on your right side and insert the tip of the enema tube into your rectum, open the spout of the enema tube and let the retention enema flow into your colon. The point is to retain the enema contents as long as possible until it soaks into the colon. Try to hold it in at least a couple of hours but if you can't, you will still be getting some healing from it.

I have also performed a retention enema with only the probiotic powders; start with a small amount and work your way up. If you start with too much probiotics in your colon, you can experience a "die-off" reaction that will give you intestinal cramps, bloating, gas, and/or burping for hours. Start with a smaller dosage and work your way up to a larger dosage.

You should also be taking probiotics internally so you are getting the intestinal benefits from both ends and re-populating your gut with good bacteria and healing the colon at the same time. However, if you have a severe leaky gut condition, make sure the probiotics are in powdered form as pills may not be effective because they can pass through the holes in the gut. Natren's is the only company I know of that carries an excellent brand of powdered probiotics that are either with or without dairy, although these probiotics can be pricey.

Now you should be feeling great with a cleansed liver. There are other methods to detoxifying the body which I will go over in latter chapters. Those who are still chronically ill after following through the colon, candida, parasite, kidney and liver cleanse, may need to repeat some of the cleanses over or it is possible that you have chronic candida infections which involve biofilm formations, you could also have other biofilm infections which are keeping you sick.

11

Biofilms

If you have attempted all the detoxes listed in this book and you still are showing little to no improvement, it may be wise to look toward biofilm infections as the possible root cause of your health issue and eradicate the biofilms in order to begin the healing process.

Biofilms are stealth infections that are impervious to antibiotics and many antifungal treatments. Biofilms consist of a slimy shell around the infections, making it difficult to break through to reach the infection or bacteria inside of the slimy shell. Biofilms will colonize and multiply if not eradicated, therefore causing further chronic disease and possibly even death if not treated. Many people who are chronically ill may have infections in the body or mouth which are caused from biofilm formations. "With an estimated 2% of the population of the United States suffering from chronic, non-healing wounds and estimates of upwards of 350 million people expected to develop diabetes by 2050, the problem of how to target bacterial biofilm effectively cannot be overestimated (Gottrup 2004; Wild et al. 2004)." (9).

"Biofilms have been found to be involved in a wide variety of microbial infections (by one estimate, 80% of all infections)." (17). Biofilms are common in chronic diseases; such as, Lyme disease, some types of candida overgrowth, MRSA, klebsiella pneumonia, pneumonia, periodontal disease, gingivitis, dental caries, peri-implantitis (infection of tooth implant), chronic sinusitis, bad breath, some ear infections, biliary tract infection, chronic fatigue syndrome, musculoskeletal infections, osteomyelitis (bone infection), fibromyalgia, coronary heart disease, native valve endocarditis (heart valve infection), necrotizing fascitis (flesh eating bacteria), legionnaire's disease, cystic fibrosis, Whitmore's disease (meloidosis), bacterial prostatitis (prostate infection), Alzheimer's disease, and dementia. The most prominent features of biofilm infections are that they are persistent and chronic in nature.

Additionally, many biofilm infections originate in hospitals and sadly many patients succumb to these infections. "In 2002, 1.7 million nosocomial bacterial infections were equivalent to an average of 4.5 infections reported for every 100-people admitted to the hospital and these infections resulted in 99,000 deaths (Klevens et al. 2007) and upwards of 65% of nosocomial infections are suspected to originate from bacterial biofilms." (9). Biofilms can be deadly if not treated properly and unfortunately, there are many doctors and dentists who are not keeping up with the latest research into treating these biofilm infections in a proper manner.

I had started looking toward biofilms as my own root cause of infections when I wasn't recovering regardless of eating an organic diet, exercising, and detoxing. Since the cancer battle I experienced in 2009 & beyond, I had also acquired extreme inflammation, severe leaky gut syndrome, advanced adrenal fatigue, auto brewery syndrome, brain fog, hormonal imbalance, advanced periodontal disease, and a tooth infection, which spread to an ear infection which wouldn't go away with antibiotics. Although, I did have the periodontal infection years prior to cancer and had felt that this infection was the main culprit behind many of my illnesses. I knew that I was sick but every doctor I went to wasn't helping and some even made me worse with their supplements and suggestions. I knew that I would have to take matters into my own hands again if I ever planned on getting well.

I had periodontal disease for many years with periodontal pockets of over 10 plus on my upper back teeth. The teeth on both upper quadrants had infections for years and the dentists never once mentioned biofilms, only removing the teeth or giving me root canals. I had attempted the gum flap surgery back in 2005, only to be told that my bone loss was significant and they weren't able to graft bone to reduce the pockets. I also declined the offer of root canals and removal of my back teeth back in 2005 and began to do oil pulling daily to try to save my teeth.

Not only was I plagued with the periodontal infection but was also harboring another biofilm infection in my gut. In February of 2014, I had a comprehensive stool analysis; ordered by a doctor, which detected the presence of klebsiella pneumonia in my stool sample. I had continued to go over my test results, deciphering each bacterium, to find out more about those bacteria and which treatment would work best. Since antibiotics are not effective in treating biofilms, it is necessary to enlist some alternative supplements that target those specific biofilms to eradicate the biofilms.

Antibiotics never worked on the tooth infections because all periodontal disease is caused from a biofilm in which antibiotics will be impervious to the infection. When I had met with another dentist about the presence of biofilms associated with periodontal disease as the primary reason that the antibiotics were not working and are resistant to that type of infection, the dentist sternly told me that "he was the expert and had never heard of biofilms." Unfortunately, this type of arrogant behavior with doctors and dentists occurs all too often because they are not doing their due diligence in keeping up with the current research in their field of study. So, I left his office knowing that I would have to heal this myself since the majority of dentists weren't going to help my condition. It wasn't until a couple of years later when I met a more qualified holistic periodontist who was familiar with biofilms and periodontal disease.

Due to the antibiotics not working to eradicate the painful tooth infection, I learned of biofilms and began experimenting on the biofilm infection in my mouth. When I began to experiment with biofilm disruptors, I used a combination of treatments to help eliminate the biofilm infections in my mouth and body, which then helped to lift the burden off of my immune system so it could do its job to begin to heal my body. It took over 5 months for the ear and tooth infection to finally clear up using 3 types of biofilm disruptors and antifungals. The pain I experienced for five months was excruciating with constant throbbing on the left side of my mouth daily which travelled all the way up to my ear canal. Once the biofilms in my mouth were eradicated, I could tell my body was slowly starting to respond to normal detoxing and food once again.

"Bacterial etiology has been confirmed for common oral diseases such as caries and periodontal and endodontic infections. Bacteria causing these diseases are organized in biofilm structures, which are complex microbial communities, composed of a great variety of bacteria with different ecological requirements and pathogenic potential. The biofilm community not only gives bacteria effective protection against the host's defense system but also makes them more resistant to a variety of disinfecting agents used as oral hygiene products or in the treatment of infections. Successful treatment of these diseases depends on biofilm removal as well as effective killing of biofilm bacteria." (10).

Many chronic diseases can be directly attributed from infections in the mouth. It has been proven that over 98% of women who have had terminal breast cancer, all had a root canal on the same tooth meridian associated with the breast. The number 2, 3, 14, and 15 teeth are directly related to the tooth/breast meridian (see figure 1). I was diagnosed with periodontal disease many years ago and oddly enough, the teeth in which I have had the most issues with infections due to periodontal disease are the number 2, 3, 14, and 15 teeth. Most recently, the number 14 tooth became really loose, on the verge of falling out regardless of the many holistic treatments I had completed to try and save my teeth. The infection was just too deep into the bone where holistic treatments and antibiotics are impervious on biofilm infections. The #14 tooth is the same meridian in which I had the breast cancer which started in my left breast back in 2009.

Although I had taken biofilm disruptors to get rid of some of the infection due to periodontal disease, I still ended up having to have the number 14 tooth removed and have additional laser treatment to treat the rest of the infections that had spread deep within the bones in my mouth. The periodontist was amazed that my tooth was hanging on so long; he said that if it were anyone else, that tooth would have fallen out long ago, but due to the treatments I continued to do, the teeth are hanging on. A few days after the laser treatment for the infection, I was feeling much better. Now, I'm sure if I had known about this information many, many years ago and started the biofilm treatments back when I was first informed of periodontal disease, I may have been able to save my tooth. My suggestion to anyone with gingivitis or beginning periodontal disease; start these biofilm and antifungal treatments early and see your dentist regularly for deep cleanings so you can save your teeth and more importantly, stave off chronic disease. Periodontal disease is also directly related to heart disease and stroke because the hardened plaque that forms around the tooth also forms around the heart valves. What both periodontal disease and heart disease have in common are the biofilm formations which cause both conditions. My good friend, who also had periodontal disease, went in for a root planing procedure, only to die of a massive heart attack hours after the oral procedure was over. I often wonder how many times people with periodontal disease die of a massive heart attack, after a major dental procedure, because the biofilm bacteria in the mouth is being disrupted by the dental procedure and that deadly bacteria can travel directly into the bloodstream and directly into the heart causing a massive heart attack or stroke. Of course, this theory can never be proven because the heart attack or stroke happens after the dental patient is already out of the dentist's chair and at home, so it is most likely chalked up to a heart attack or stroke with no connection ever being made to the dental procedure, disrupting the biofilm, which happened earlier.

Alternatively, when someone has a root canal procedure, the dentist removes the root and fills the tooth, but the infection is left in the bone to spread and eventually may cause cancer and/or other diseases. On the next page, you will find the tooth meridian chart that gives you information on which teeth are correlated with which organ/disease.

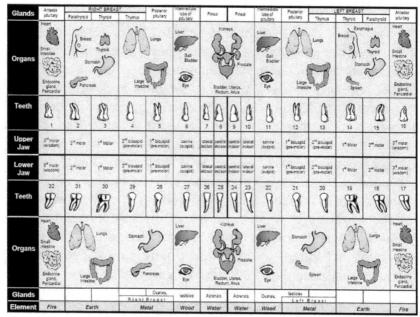

Figure 12: www.holisticdentist.com

Those who currently have periodontal disease, you have a biofilm infection and you need to get rid of the biofilm immediately before it leads to cancer and other diseases. Most importantly, you already have had or currently have chronic disease, which may be caused by a biofilm. If you do not eradicate the biofilm, chronic disease will continue to progress.

There are some natural treatments which can help to irrigate the root canal or periodontal area and will help the most if you are still in the early stages of gingivitis. I prefer Nature's Answer PerioBrite and Nature's Answer PerioCleanse. The PerioCleanse is a concentrated cleansing solution that can be pumped into a waterpik device and used to irrigate and treat infections. The PerioBrite is used as a mouthwash after brushing. Both of these products do contain plant derivatives that target biofilm formations; such as, clove bud oil (eugenol) and Berberine (Goldenseal). Although, I have used the internal biofilm agents to heal infection, I also use the oral agents daily to keep the infections at bay for a while. These treatments will obviously have a better effect on those in which the infection hasn't already spread deep into the bone.

"Plant-derived natural products represent a rich source of antimicrobial compounds, and some have been incorporated into oral hygiene products. However, their application in endodontics is less well documented. Berberine is an alkaloid present in a number of clinically important medicinal plants, including goldenseal, Coptis chinensis (coptis or golden thread), and others. It possesses a broad antimicrobial spectrum against bacteria, fungi, protozoans, virus, helminths, and chlamydia." (10).

What you will notice when you are breaking through the biofilms in your body successfully: If the biofilm is in your mouth, as in periodontal disease, your teeth will ache considerably and throb with intense pain all throughout the day. You will be able to tell which type of biofilm infection you have, based upon which treatment works. For instance, whenever I took a biofilm disruptor that targets candida, my teeth would have intense pain and throbbing, so I knew that the biofilm was being disrupted. If I took a biofilm disruptor that targeted the klebsiella pneumonia in my gut, my teeth wouldn't hurt. If you have any chronic infection that is biofilm related, there are certain herbal supplements that help to break through biofilms.

Biofilm Disruptors:

There are specific herbal supplements that will only break through the slimy outer shell of the biofilm. Using traditional herbal antifungals geared toward candida or parasites will not work as most of those are not strong enough to break through the biofilm, although they work great to target the candida and parasite once you have broken through the biofilm layer. I have experienced the most success with using the biofilm disruptors first and then waiting about an hour and then taking anti-fungals and/or anti-parasitics to target the infection, candida, or parasite more effectively.

It is best to take these biofilm disruptors on an empty stomach and approximately 30-60 minutes prior to the antifungals for biofilms. These biofilm disruptors will break through the wall of the biofilm to open it up so the anti-fungal can target the infection. Not all of these biofilm disruptors will work for you, it depends upon the type of biofilm that you have. It is also best to combine these biofilm disruptors together to get the most effective biofilm disruptor. At least three biofilm disruptors should be combined, as this is proven to be the most effective. Everyone will be different and the combinations will not work for everyone. It would be best to find a knowledgeable doctor who knows about eradicating biofilms and healing naturally, although finding a doctor with this knowledge has proven to be very difficult. So, if you find you are not healing with using anti-fungals alone for candida and herbals for parasites, you may need to add the biofilm disruptors as well.

I suggest continuing coffee enemas and/or other methods of supporting the liver throughout the process of disrupting and killing off biofilms to flush the amount of toxins being released into the liver to avoid re-intoxicating your body with harmful toxins. The following is a list of the biofilm disrupting supplements.

Biofilm Disrupting Supplements:

Choose three biofilm disruptors based upon your individual symptoms or health issue. Combine the three and then wait 30-60 minutes before taking the anti-fungals to target infection.

Klaire Labs Interfase Plus (EDTA): "Biofilms consist of groups of bacteria attached to surfaces and encased in a hydrated polymeric matrix. Bacteria in biofilms are more resistant to the immune system and to antibiotics than their free-living planktonic counterparts. Thus, biofilm-related infections are persistent and often show recurrent symptoms. The metal chelator EDTA is known to have activity against biofilms of gram-positive bacteria such as Staphylococcus aureus. EDTA can also kill planktonic cells of Proteobacteria like Pseudomonas aeruginosa." (8).

EDTA is successful in breaking through biofilms of Klebsiella pneumonia, Pseudomonas, Staphylococcus epidermidis, Staphylococcus aureus, and Candida albicans. "EDTA facilitates biofilm detachment and lysis." (8). Lysis is the process of the

128

breaking down of the cell. "Chen and Stewart have previously tested the abilities of various chemical treatments to remove mixed P. aeruginosa-Klebsiella pneumoniae biofilms. They reported that EDTA treatment resulted in a 49% reduction in cell counts, and they presented some evidence that this was due to dispersal of biofilm bacteria." (12). From the Journal of Applied and Environmental Microbiology, the use of "EDTA causes detachment and killing of biofilm cells." (8).

When I first started taking EDTA in the form of Interfase Plus, I was taking 8 pills per day and it was making me very tired, which all biofilm disruptors will do if you have a biofilm present, because it was detoxing the biofilm in my body too fast. I had to reduce my dosage to 2-4 pills per day to make the detoxing symptoms more manageable.

At first, the EDTA (Interfase Plus) made me feel horrible but as I improved, it didn't make me feel bad any longer. This of course was after I had been taking it for over 5 months. Start slowly with the biofilm disruptors so you are not releasing the biofilms too quickly and causing a re-intoxication issue.

Thorne Laboratories SF722: This is made from 10-undecenoic acid and is derived from the castor plant, which is used to make castor oil. SF722 is used for Candida biofilms and periodontal disease. This is stronger than caprylic acid for Candida infections.

Serrapepidase or Serrapeptase: For Lyme disease, Borrelia bacteria, lung function, silk worm, tick infections, and staphylococcus aureus. Serrapeptase is derived from the digestive tract of a silk worm. It is a Proteolytic enzyme, which comes from a species of gut bacteria found in the intestines of the silkworm. Serrapeptase is known to break through certain biofilm formations and cancerous tumors to help aid in healing the body of inflammation. The reason it breaks through cancerous tumors is because cancer cells are coated with a protein layer that needs to be penetrated to reach the inner core of the cancer cell.

Serrapeptase digests dead tissue in the arteries and digestive tract and also has anti-inflammatory properties.

Serrapeptase is good for dissolving blood clots, plaque along the arterial wall, infections of the ear, nose, throat, lung congestion, asthma, diabetes, ulcers, and easing inflammation.

Serrapeptase should be taken in increments of 20,000 IU or more. This is where it is beneficial to have a knowledgeable doctor to help to gauge the dosage. I have personally not found many doctors who are knowledgeable regarding biofilms, much less on how much serrapeptase to take. I have personally taken up to 240,000 IUs per day, which may have been too much as the side effect was a consistent phlegm type cough. When I reduced the dosage to only 120,000 IUs, the cough went away.

Lumbrokinase: An enzyme produced by earthworms which is known to dissolve the fibrin coating of the biofilm. Used to dissolve Borrelia bacteria associated with Lyme disease. May also help those with Alzheimer's and Dementia whose root cause may be Lyme disease.

Nattokinase: derived from the Japanese fermented soybean meal called Natto. Nattokinase is an enzyme with fibrinolytic activity, which can break through the fibrin of the biofilms and help with Alzheimer's, Dementia, hypertension, and retinal disorders.

Lactoferrin: "Candida albicans, as well as a number of bacterial species including the opportunistic pathogen Pseudomonas aeruginosa (van der Kraan et al. 2004)." (9). Klebsiella, Candida "Lactoferrin is an abundant, iron-binding protein from the innate immune system (reviewed in Valenti et al. 2004) found circulating in the blood, as well as in secreted fluids such as tears, semen, vaginal secretions, and most recently sweat (Park et al. 2011). Found in greatest abundance in milk, lactoferrin is generally thought of as a milk protein. However, lactoferrin is a multifunctional protein serving many roles." (9).

"In addition to being anti-inflammatory, lactoferrin has demonstrated anti-tumor, anti-viral, anti-fungal, and anti-bacterial properties (Farnaud & Evans 2003)." (9). "The most obvious mechanism of lactoferrin action is that by binding and sequestering the iron in the environment, lactoferrin deprives the biofilm of this essential nutrient, thus limits the capacity of the biofilm to survive." (9).

"Lactoferrin therapy is effective against infections of the urinary tract and lactoferrin has been used as an oral treatment for irritable bowel syndrome with a normalizing effect on the gut microbiome (Bellamy et al. 1993; Zagulski et al. 1998; Ha & Kornbluth 2010; Hu et al. 2012; Ochoa et al. 2012)." (9).

Colloidal Silver: For Staphylococcus aureus, chronic rhinosinusitis. "Treatment of recalcitrant chronic rhinosinusitis (CRS) is a challenge with increasing antibiotic resistance, leading to re-emergence of topical therapies." (11). Colloidal Silver was used as a flush of the frontal sinus and found to be effective at killing the biofilm associated with sinusitis and staphylococcus aureus. I have also used colloidal silver as a rinse in my PerioBrite mouthwash as well as adding it to my waterpik for helping to eradicate infection caused from periodontal infection.

Garlic (Allicin): Allicin is effective at eradicating all biofilms, although Allicin is less effective at disrupting biofilms when it is heated. (18). Allicin is effective against biofilm strains of Staphylococcus epidermidis. (16). Allicin also works against Candida Albicans and Pseudomonas.

Clove (Eugenol): For periodontal disease, Klebsiella pneumonia, and Candida Albicans. Eugenol is found in many essential oils with the highest concentration of eugenol being found in cloves and some eugenol being found in cinnamon. Eugenol also can cause breast cancer cell death. (18). "Candida albicans is the most frequently isolated causative pathogen of candidiasis and the biofilms display significantly increased levels of resistance to the conventional antifungal agents. Eugenol, the major phenolic component of clove essential oil, possesses potent antifungal activity." (12). "Eugenol displayed potent activity against C. albicans biofilms in vitro with low cytotoxicity and therefore has potential therapeutic implication for biofilm-associated candida infections." (12).

"Natural compounds such as eugenol with anti-microbial properties are attractive agents that could reduce the use of conventional antibiotics. This study demonstrated that eugenol exhibits notable activity against MRSA and MSSA clinical strains biofilms. Eugenol inhibited biofilm formation, disrupted the cell-to-cell connections, detached the existing biofilms, and killed the bacteria in biofilms of both MRSA and MSSA with equal effectiveness. Therefore, eugenol may be used to control or eradicate S. aureus biofilm-related infections." (13).

Xylitol: Xylitol is a sugar alcohol that helps to diminish oral biofilms and wounds. "In vitro analysis of combined treatment with Xylitol and lactoferrin of the opportunistic pathogen P. aeruginosa suggested that Xylitol and lactoferrin act synergistically against P. aeruginosa grown as a biofilm. While lactoferrin destabilizes the membrane, allowing Xylitol to cross the bacterial membrane more effectively." (9).

If you have Xylitol at home, you can take 1 teaspoon into your mouth and begin swishing it around with your saliva for at least 5 minutes. Once you spit the mixture out, do not rinse your mouth but let the Xylitol go to work on any biofilm formations in your mouth.

Erythritol: Erythritol is a sugar alcohol, found to be superior to Xylitol or Sorbitol, which helps to diminish oral biofilms and wounds. "Xylitol preferentially targeted P. aeruginosa, while erythritol preferentially targeted both P. aeruginosa and S. aureus." (14).

Stevia: Stevia is a plant that is a natural replacement for sugar. This is used for dental biofilms, as "Stevia was able to drop the number of living biofilm-protected bacteria." (18). It did not eliminate the biofilm bacteria in the mouth completely, but it did reduce the dental damage. (18).

Cumunda: Cumunda comes from a tree located in the Amazon in Peru. It is available in tincture or capsule form from Nutramedix. (18). Cumunda works for killing the biofilms of Bartonella and Lyme.

Manuka Honey: Used for chronic sinusitis and deep nose infections. Manuka honey has an active component called methylglyoxal (MGO) which demonstrates anti-biofilm activity.

Be careful with the manuka honey if using it as sinus irrigation because a 50% concentration of the manuka honey did have bacteria killing actions against biofilms of pseudomonas aeruginosa and staphylococcus aureus, but this concentration also causes severe or intense inflammation that can produce facial paralysis, vestibulotixicity, and hearing loss in the chinchillas that were tested upon. (18). However, using the manuka honey in a dietary manner may still help, without the side effects.

Gingerol: Derived from ginger, Gingerol has an anti-bacterial, anti-inflammatory, and anti-tumor effect in pancreatic cancer. (18).

Anti-fungals to Target Biofilm Infections:

These anti-fungals are to be taken 30 to 60 minutes after taking the biofilm disruptor. The reason for waiting a period of time is that you want to open the slimy shell of the biofilm first with the biofilm disruptor and then target the inside of that shell with the anti-fungal to kill the infection, bacteria, candida, etc. If you experience too much pain with taking these, reduce the dosage or start out slow and increase as the infection gets better. You can combine these as well but realize that the stronger it is, the more pain and discomfort you may feel. Make sure to do the coffee enemas or other methods of supporting the liver to flush the liver of toxins. Many of these are also used to eradicate candida, bacteria, viruses, and parasites.

Oregano Oil: Wild Oregano Oil is an anti-inflammatory, anti-viral, anti-bacterial, anti-fungal, and anti-parasitic. Wild Oregano is grown wild in the Mediterranean. (19). The active ingredient of Wild Oregano is Carvacrol, which has been found to reduce infection as effectively as traditional antibiotics. I have been using oregano oil for years and North American Spice Company Wild Oregano Oil has a high carvacrol level. Studies have found that Wild Oregano Oil does kill a few parasites in some people. (21). It is mostly used for Candida and other infections. However, it does work great to keep bacteria at bay and you should always have a bottle of this in your medicine cabinet or carry it with you when you go out. There is also oregano juice to take by the tablespoon full and oregano pills.

Garlic: Containing Allicin, which is what gives garlic its odor, is also what makes garlic an anti-viral, anti-bacterial, and anti-fungal. Garlic also contains sulphur, arginine, oligosaccharides, flavonoids, and selenium, all of which may be beneficial to health. (23). Garlic has also been studied as an anti-cancer compound, "Several population studies show an association between increased intake of garlic and reduced risk of certain cancers, including cancers of the stomach, colon, esophagus, pancreas, and breast." (23).

"The World Health Organization's (WHO) guidelines for general health promotion for adults is a daily dose of 2 to 5 g of fresh garlic (approximately one clove), 0.4 to 1.2 g of dried garlic powder, 2 to 5 mg of garlic oil, 300 to 1,000 mg of garlic extract, or other formulations that are equal to 2 to 5 mg of Allicin." (23). I have found that it is easiest to take in odorless Garlic pills or if you want to prepare the fresh garlic; I blend one clove of garlic, 1 thumbful of ginger and water and drink it down really quick. It doesn't taste good, but it sure packs a powerful health tonic.

Garlic is a natural blood thinner, so those who are on blood thinning medication should be cautious with using Garlic. (23). Another powerful brand of Allicin is called Allimax, although quite expensive.

Tanalbit: a zinc tannate which works very well for acetaldehyde type candida infections, but go very slow with the dosage as this is very strong. It contains dry heated milk so may be a problem for those with milk allergies or lactose intolerance.

Tanalbit helps with a healthy digestion; it works as an antioxidant and may help in the detoxification process. (24). I have found that if you do not have candida overgrowth, this formula will not bother you. If you have extensive candida overgrowth in the digestive tract or bloodstream, this is a very strong product and should be eased into gently. I used this in combination when healing auto brewery syndrome in my bloodstream and leaky gut.

Linalool: For Candida albicans, lactobacillus casei, staphylococcus aureus, streptococcus sobrinus and mutans, gingivalis. (18). Linalool means "wood of aloe" and is often used in soap making and perfumes as it has a nice smell. Linalool is most effective when the essential oil is used. (18). This does help remove some biofilms, but did not remove biofilms formed by "Staphylococcus aureus and Escherichia coli on surfaces of medical materials; such as urinary catheters, infusion tubes and surgical mesh." (18).

Cats Claw: Cat's Claw comes from the Peruvian Rainforest. Cat's Claw is used for "tumors and other growths, ulcers, gastritis, arthritis, rheumatism, menstrual disorders, prostate problems, asthma, diabetes, viral infections, gonorrhea, cirrhosis, general debility, bursitis, genital herpes, herpes zoster, allergies, systemic candidiasis, PMS, environmental toxin poisoning, bowel and intestinal disorders, organic depression and HIV infection." (25).

Wormwood: Used for parasitic activity to target the adult parasites. Wormwood is originally known as Artemisia, which is the key ingredient in Absinthe. (26). Wormwood is useful to keep insects and parasites away, but "The bitter components and acids render wormwood an excellent remedy for digestive issues. This is primarily because a bitter flavor on the tongue actually causes the gallbladder to produce and release bile." (26). Taking too much wormwood can cause diarrhea. (26).

Oregon Grape: "Oregon grape root contains berberine, also found in barberry, coptis, and goldenseal. The herb also contains phytochemicals with similar activity, including columbamine, hydrastine, jatrorrhizine, oxyacanthine, and tetrahydroberberine, as well as tannins." (27). Oregon grape is very similar to goldenseal. "It is also traditionally used as a bitter tonic to stimulate digestion and externally for its antimicrobial properties. The active constituents in Oregon grape root have shown substantial antimicrobial and antifungal activity in vitro, though these activities are unproven in human trials." (27).

Oregon grape has a high level of berberine and Vitamin C and works as an anti-biotic, an astringent, alterative, diuretic and it works well as a laxative. It has the ability to stimulate a thyroid, which makes it a good option for those that have an inactive or under producing thyroid. It is helpful in treating fevers, upset stomachs, scurvy, reduces sore throats and boosts the immune system. (28). It can also be used topically to treat acne, abrasions, eczema, psoriasis and similar conditions. To use it for this reason, a small dab of the Oregon grape root extract is applied to the area. (28).

Goldenseal: Goldenseal is an herbal anti-biotic, anti-inflammatory, astringent, and immune system enhancer. "Goldenseal contains calcium, iron, manganese, vitamin A, vitamin C, vitamin E, B-complex, and other nutrients and minerals." (26). The primary alkaloid in Goldenseal is Berberine which is why it is effective against bacteria, protozoa, fungi, Streptococci, anti-bacterial, and anti-fungal. (26).

It has been used as a medication for inflammatory conditions; such as respiratory, digestive and genito-urinary tract inflammation induced by allergy or infection. (26).

"It soothes irritated mucus membranes helping the eyes, ears, nose and throat. Goldenseal works for respiratory problems, colds or flu, when taken at the first sign of these issues. It has also been used to help reduce fevers, and relieve congestion and excess mucous." (26).

"Goldenseal cleanses and promotes healthy glandular functions by increasing bile flow and digestive enzymes, therefore regulating healthy liver and spleen functions. It can relieve constipation and may also be used to treat infections of the bladder and intestines as well as help with allergic rhinitis, hay fever, laryngitis, hepatitis, cystitis, and alcoholic liver disease, eczema, ringworm, excessive menstruation, internal bleeding, wounds, earaches, gum infections, sore throat, boils, abscesses, and carbuncles." (26). Goldenseal can be used as a wash, drops, and a poultice for multiple uses previously mentioned.

Grapefruit Seed Extract: "All over the world, Grapefruit Seed Extract (GSE) has been used for killing a wide variety of bacteria (such as: Salmonella, E. coli, Staph and Strep germs), viruses, herpes, parasites, and fungi, including Candida. It is effective against more than 800 bacterial and viral strains, 100 strains of fungus, as well as a large number of single-cell and multi-celled parasites. It has also proven to be effective against food poisoning and diarrhea."

You can also use any of the anti-fungals in the Candida chapter to target the yeast, bacteria, fungus after breaking open the biofilm.

What to Use to Flush the Toxins:

A few hours after taking the biofilm disruptor and then the anti-fungals, I would do coffee enemas to flush the liver and take one or more of the following to help bind the toxins that are being released from the body. Of course, it all depends upon how you are feeling as the coffee enema will help to flush the liver of the excess toxins so you don't overburden your liver or re-introduce toxins into your body. So, a few of these will help your body to cart out the toxins from the biofilms; such as spirulina, chlorella, liquid bentonite clay and psyllium husk.

Other supplements; such as, N-Acetyl cysteine (NAC), N-Acetyl glucosamine (NAG), and colostrum will help to reduce inflammation and boost the immune system. It is important to boost your immune system during the detoxification process to help your body to work as it is supposed to. When you are healthy, your immune system helps to fight off disease on its own. When you are ill, it is important to take these immune boosting supplements to help your body repair and be able to fight off inflammation and illness.

Spirulina: Spirulina is blue - green algae and is found in lakes, ponds, and rivers. Spirulina is rich in iron, magnesium and trace minerals, and is easier to absorb than iron supplements. Spirulina is the highest source of B-12 and contains more beta carotene than carrots. (30). The phytonutrients in spirulina include chlorophyll, phycocyanin and polysaccharides, which can help cleanse the toxins from our bodies. (30).

Spirulina is high in Gamma linolenic acid (GLA), which is a compound found in breast milk to help develop healthier babies. Spirulina can also help the body absorb nutrients when the body has lost its ability to absorb normal forms of food. It stimulates beneficial flora of lactobacillus and bifidobacteria and promotes healthy digestion and regular bowel function. (30).

Spirulina is a natural detoxifier for heavy metals and other deadly toxins. It also contains the nutrients of iron, manganese, zinc, copper, selenium, and chromium, which help to fight free radicals. These nutrients can also help the immune system to fight cancer and cellular degeneration. (30).

I personally take spirulina every morning in a smoothie (see recipe in leaky gut chapter). It makes it much easier to just add spirulina powder to a smoothie as opposed to taking yet another pill. I also took extra spirulina after having all of my mercury fillings removed at the dentist office. I took spirulina before going into the dentist that morning of the procedure and after coming out and for a few days afterward to make sure to soak up any mercury toxicity that the dentist may have missed.

Chlorella: Similar to Spirulina, Chlorella is also a fresh water algae which helps to detoxify the body. It helps to boost the immune system to help fight infections. Chlorella increases good bacteria in the gastrointestinal tract, treats ulcers, colitis, diverticulitis, and Crohn's disease. Chlorella protects the body from cancerous radiation treatments, treats constipation, high blood pressure, diabetes, asthma, fibromyalgia, and high cholesterol. (31). The abundance of Chlorophyll in the Chlorella is what protects the body against ultraviolet radiation. (31).

Liquid Bentonite Clay: has a positive charge which attracts the negative charge of toxic material to cart it out of the body. I prefer the yerba prima Great Plains brand of liquid bentonite clay, which is already pre-mixed for you and very easy to take without any taste.

I take the liquid bentonite clay with a few ounces of the clay in a small glass and then follow it up with a full glass of room temperature water. The room temperature water will help the bentonite clay to expand and soak up all of the toxins along the way from the mouth to the anus.

Psyllium husk (if you don't have leaky gut): This is best taken at night to help bind the toxins and also to scrub the digestive tract of toxic debris and cart it out of the body. Although the psyllium husk method may be too harsh or not work at all for those with leaky gut. In which case, you must heal the gut lining first before using psyllium husk. Refer back to the colon cleanse chapter for instructions on how to do this properly.

You can also use fresh ground flaxseeds in place of psyllium husk. If you can't handle either the psyllium husk or ground flaxseeds, you can just use the liquid bentonite clay portion of this cleanse.

Activated Charcoal: This binds to the toxins and carts them out of the body. However, it is not safe to use more than a couple of days a week. I have taken 3 – 5 activated charcoal capsules with a full glass of room temperature water with each pill. These charcoal capsules will constipate you, so make sure to drink plenty of water. Also, this will turn your stool black so don't be alarmed the next time you go to the toilet.

N-Acetyl Cysteine (NAC): NAC comes from the amino acid L-cysteine. This is normally used to counteract the toxic effects of acetaminophen (Tylenol). NAC is a precursor to glutathione, which detoxifies the body from free radicals, helps to repair cell damage and boosts the immune system. (32/33).

N-Acetyl Glucosamine (NAG): N-acetyl glucosamine (NAG) is a monosaccharide derivative of glucose. NAG can correct an overactive immune system so that autoimmune reactions occur less often. The mechanisms of action believed to be behind correcting an overactive immune system is that NAG controls immune T-cell over activity and stabilizes mast cells. (34).

NAG is also involved in the repair of mucous membranes throughout the body. NAG helps to decrease inflammation and is known as a natural remedy for Irritable Bowel Disease,

Crohn's disease, Multiple Sclerosis, Osteoarthritis, and Ulcerative Colitis. (35). It also decreases the binding of some lectins (proteins that may damage the intestines) from food ingestion. NAG helps to correctly regulate your gut flora by maintaining the mucosal barrier and preventing Small Intestinal Bacterial Overgrowth (SIBO) from occurring. (34).

Colostrum: derived from the milk of the cow, "this superfood creates no problems for those with lactose intolerance." (37). Colostrum helps to re-build the immune system for those with compromised immune systems. Colostrum can help to reduce the time you are sick with a cold or flu and is more effective than any flu shot. (36).

Colostrum has been proven to improve lean muscle tissue growth; it improves muscle recovery, and reduces soreness so this is a perfect supplement for athletes. (36). Since colostrum is an anti-inflammatory, it is excellent for reducing pain and inflammation from arthritis, colitis, chronic fatigue syndrome, fibromyalgia, multiple sclerosis, rheumatoid arthritis, lupus, scleraderma and other inflammatory conditions.

"Tumor necrosis factor-alpha (TNF-a) is found in Colostrum, and this substance helps to effectively "turn off" the inflammation at the source. Another helpful ingredient is interleukin-1ra (IL-1ra), a protein that helps to reduce inflammation caused by certain conditions. Not only does IL-1ra contain helpful substances to reduce swelling and pain, but it's been shown to aid in cases of chronic inflammatory diseases, like arthritis and Crohn's disease. Proline rich peptides (PRPs) are also found in Colostrum, and these act as an oxidative stress regulator." (36).

Colostrum also helps relieve your allergies and reduces asthma symptoms. Allergies in human beings are caused by Immunoglobulin E (IgE), which is produced the body as a response to a foreign protein that enters the body. Colostrum can actually help desensitize your body to these allergens by helping to lower the expression of IgE. Since Colostrum has a high concentration of antibodies, it can help your body fight off allergies and suppress its reaction to the allergens that do make it through.

Another added benefit of Colostrum is that it helps with Alzheimer's disease and other cognitive disorders by reducing the severity of the disease. In a clinical trial including Colostrum and a placebo, all of the participants in the study had Alzheimer's disease, over 50% of the participants who received Colostrum showed clinical improvement, and the rest of them stabilized; those who received only a placebo did not show any improvement. Phosphatidylserine is the substance found in high concentrations in Colostrum supplements which is why it has shown to be of help to those who suffer from Alzheimer's or senile dementia. (36).

Colostrum also includes high amounts of antioxidants; including glutathione, which is the master detoxifier mentioned in the chapter on liver detox. The Antioxidants in the Colostrum fights against aging and can help you to look younger. (36).

The most important point to take away from this chapter is that biofilms can be deadly if not eradicated. Unfortunately, many will not find help with their local doctor as their knowledge of biofilms are limited at best. Therefore, it is imperative to first target the biofilm before targeting the specific infection within the biofilm formation. Many of you may not have a chronic or extreme condition that contains a biofilm, in which case the normal detoxing methods should work fine on their own.

12

Juice Fasting

Another method of detoxifying the body is through a juice fast, where you give your digestive system a rest and subsist on nothing more than freshly prepared juices and raw blended soups daily. Juice fasting is a good way to accomplish the colon cleanse, candida cleanse, parasite cleanse, kidney cleanse, and liver cleanse all at the same time depending upon the vegetables, fruits, and herbs that you juice.

There are different theories on the best method to complete a juice fast; through juicing or blending fruits and vegetables. Juicing will press the juice from the fruits or vegetables, leaving only the juice and eliminating the pulp from the fruit or vegetable. This is a good method but can also become very expensive because you will yield little juice in comparison to the amount of fruits and vegetables being used. Since juicing produces only the juice, it will be absorbed into your cells quicker. Juicing may cause constipation, due to the lack of fiber pushing the toxic waste through the colon. In which case, it may be necessary to perform an enema to help to eliminate the waste.

Blending the fruits and vegetables, in a high-speed blender, will keep the pulp and fiber within the juice; also known as smoothies. With the fiber intact, your colon will stay in the game and you will be less constipated. The blended fruits and vegetables will retain the fiber to help eliminate toxic waste, but you may still need to perform an enema on occasion.

Which method is better, juicing or blending, is dependent upon your preference and current state of health. I personally like blending the fruits and vegetables because it retains the fiber and yields more juice, so I save money in the long run. I also make sure to perform coffee enemas to help to detoxify my liver at the same time as detoxifying my colon and other organs in my body.

As was stated by Dr. Norman Walker; "Vegetable juices are the builders and regenerators of the body. They contain all the amino acids minerals, salts, enzymes, and vitamins needed by the human body provided that they are used fresh, raw, and without preservatives and that they have been properly extracted from the vegetables." (5).

Juicing is where the juice from a vegetable or fruit is extracted from the pulp, leaving only the juice. A masticating type juicer or blender will blend the entire vegetable or fruit, leaving the pulp within the juice (smoothie). Different types of juicers available on the market are; Omega, Champion, Jack LaLane, Hurom, Breville juice fountain, and many others. Different types of Masticating Blenders on the market are the; Vitamix, Blendtec, and Montel Williams. It is based upon personal preference as to which one will work best for you.

I personally use a Vitamix blender and also an Omega HRT standing juicer, because Vitamix is high powered and easy to clean. I also chose the Omega HRT juicer because it is the easiest to clean and I couldn't be happier. If your juicer or blender is not easy to clean, you may not be as willing to change your dietary habits. I now use both my juicer and blender on a regular basis.

The Benefits of Vegetable Juices:

The benefits of vegetable juices are that the juice can assimilate into the body quicker because there is no fiber to digest. With juicing, you are giving your digestive system a much needed rest to heal and repair itself, while still getting all of the vitamins, enzymes, and minerals you need within the juice. This is a definite benefit to juicing over blending. However, juicing can be very costly because you have to use a large amount of vegetables to get a small amount of juice. I like juicing, but I could not afford it while I was healing cancer naturally, so I opted for vegetable smoothies instead so the majority of the vegetable wouldn't be wasted and I would drink the pulp.

The Benefits of Vegetable Smoothies:

A vegetable smoothie is a combination of vegetables blended with a high-powered blender, strong enough to pulverize anything that goes into it, called a masticating blender. The benefit of a vegetable smoothie, as opposed to green juice, is that a smoothie leaves the pulp within the juice and is therefore a great method of detoxification and can also be used for a juice fast, which is a great way to detoxify the colon and other organs in the body.

Some people may suffer from intestinal permeability (leaky gut) issues due to the toxins, chemotherapy, radiation, or antibiotics which have altered their gut flora. Drinking smoothies may be too difficult for those with intestinal permeability to digest the pulp from the raw vegetables. Therefore, it may be necessary to use a juicer at first to help to replace the lost minerals within the body, without the added strain of trying to digest the fibers from the vegetables. When I had severe leaky gut, I had problems with all raw foods including raw vegetable juices, and my body just couldn't absorb or tolerate any of the raw vegetables in any form. Again, which works best for you is based on personal opinion and the current state of your health. Try both and see which one works best for you.

If you only have a high-powered blender; such as a Vitamix, Blendtec or Nutribullet and cannot afford a juicer but would like to try juice, You can always use a nut milk bag, muslin bag, or fine mesh strainer and pour your blended vegetables into the bag squeezing all of the pulp in the bag and squeezing the juice into a bowl or glass. You can then pour the extracted juice into a glass and enjoy. You can then use the leftover pulp, which has been drained of the juice, to make into vegetable patties, put them into a meatloaf, make up some baby food, or add a bit of the pulp to your pet's food so they can experience increased nutrition as well. You can get a very good nut milk bag on Amazon for a reasonable price.

If you feel that you need help in your healing process and want to learn more about juicing for health, the Gerson clinic, located in San Diego, CA and Baja California, is a great alternative to learn how to juice and heal the body naturally.

Gerson Therapy:

Dr. Max Gerson, a medical doctor from Germany, had begun using metabolic therapy to heal many "incurable" diseases. Although he had first set up a medical practice in 1919 in Germany, he had immigrated to the United States in 1936 to set up his medical practice in New York. Dr. Gerson's therapy utilized many vegetable juices throughout the day, supplements, and coffee enemas. Those who have utilized Dr. Gerson's therapy of drinking vegetable juices and practicing coffee enemas, have healed from many diseases, including cancer.

Dr. Gerson, like many other doctors who heal cancer and other diseases naturally, was referred to as a quack by the medical establishment. And even though he had written books and published over 50 papers regarding his findings, the American Medical Association and the National Cancer Institute refused to look at his successful treatment for cancer and other diseases. He eventually lost his license to practice medicine in the state of New York and moved his practice to California, where it still sits today.

The Gerson Institute, located in San Diego, CA. with a clinic in Tijuana, Mexico, is run by Dr. Max Gerson's daughter, Charlotte Gerson. Charlotte practices her father's successful treatment for cancer and other diseases and people from all over the world flock to the Gerson center for treatment. The Gerson treatment utilizes 13 fresh pressed juices daily, from only organically grown fruits and vegetables. Five coffee enemas per day are used to help cleanse the liver of toxins. The patients are also put on a strict diet with no salts, no sugars, and very little meats. The Gerson method also utilizes supplements within their therapy.

While I was healing cancer naturally, I only utilized portions of the Gerson method due to the high cost of the supplements. I only juiced 3 times per day and maintained a very strict diet. I did not start utilizing coffee enemas until after the second time I had cancer, but I was detoxifying my body and was using Dr.

Hulda Clark's method of detoxifying the liver; which you will find in the chapter on liver detoxification.

Which Vegetables to Juice:

Your personal health challenges will determine which fruits or vegetables are best to use. If you have cancer, you will want to stay away from too many fruits that are high in sugar content because cancer feeds on sugar. Also, too many sweet fruits or vegetables can also raise blood sugar, causing blood sugar imbalances. So, it would be best to stick with vegetables that are low in sugar. It is always best to juice raw vegetables and fruits separately and not mix the two, but it is understandable that when you are new to juicing that you may need to add a few slices of apple for sweetness. It is also imperative to rotate the fruits and vegetables, so you are not overloading on one specific vegetable or fruit every time you make a juice or smoothie.

The basics of most juicing recipes, and some of my favorites include, spinach, kale, celery, cucumber, carrots, apples, parsley, romaine, red bell pepper, ginger and beets. You can start with these to begin with and then experiment with other fruits and vegetables.

Help, I've Turned Orange:

Juicing carrots are very beneficial for cancer and other diseases due to the beta carotene properties, which carry a live electrical charge, and are cleansing to the liver. According to Dr. Norman Walker, "Raw carrot juice is a natural solvent for ulcerous and cancerous conditions." (5). Mostly all cancer patients and people who are chronically ill have a clogged liver and when you juice carrots, it will cleanse the liver and sometimes will discolor your skin a yellowish/orange tint. The reason that the carrots have this effect is not due to the beta carotene in the carrot, but that the liver is clogged and is getting a much needed cleansing. So, be thankful if you turn orange as this means that your body and liver is cleansing itself. The orange/yellow tint will dissipate eventually. (5).

Goitrogenic Foods:

Those people who are diagnosed with hypothyroidism or low thyroid should not juice certain raw fruits and vegetables in copious amounts because it will suppress the thyroid function further, causing extreme weight gain. (3). If you currently have low thyroid or hypothyroid, please use the goitrogenic fruits or vegetables on a rotation and sparingly. If you do not have a thyroid issue, then you can safely juice raw vegetables and fruits, but I still suggest rotating them.

You can still juice or make smoothies in its raw state, or you can also steam the vegetables first to remove the goitrogenic properties and then also drink the juice that the vegetables were steamed in so you don't lose the vitamin and mineral content. I usually add the steamed juice directly into my Vitamix to make my green smoothies or raw soups. I also still juice raw vegetables but now rotate the goitrogens.

The reason that I had learned about goitrogens was because I had a negative reaction from juicing too many goitrogenic greens at once. By January of 2011, after my second bout with cancer in December of 2010 and God saving me from certain death, I had enough energy back to start vegetable smoothies again and was drinking around 100 ounces per day of spinach and kale smoothies. I couldn't figure out why I kept gaining 10 lbs. per month, when I was on a juice fast and hiking 50 miles per week. After 5 months and 50 lbs. of excess weight gain, I figured that I had low thyroid and went to a doctor to confirm the diagnosis. I was diagnosed with low thyroid, although, it was a no-brainer, as I could tell that I already had a thyroid condition from the extreme symptoms I had experienced and the diagnosis just confirmed what I already knew.

One of my downfalls is that I do not know the word; Moderation. With me, it is all or nothing and juicing that much spinach and kale, without rotating my vegetables, had caused extreme weight gain because it further blocked thyroid production which was already low due to the leaky gut, candida, parasites, and chronic illness. There is nothing more horrible than gaining weight from vegetables because everyone assumes that I must sit around eating fattening foods, when in fact, my diet was better than most.

My advice to you is to please rotate your vegetables and don't go overboard with any one vegetable, but use moderation. The following is a list of goitrogenic foods that should be used sparingly and rotated often, especially if you have a thyroid condition. Although some of these foods on the list should never be ingested due to being genetically modified as well as being goitrogen:

Goitrogenic Food List:

- Alfalfa sprouts
- Anything with soy
- Bamboo shoots
- Broccoli
- Brussel sprouts
- Cabbage
- Canola
- Canola oil
- Cauliflower
- Collard greens
- Kale
- Kohlrabi
- Millet
- Mustard
- Mustard greens
- Peanuts
- Pears
- Pine nuts
- Peaches
- Radishes
- Rutabagas
- Soy
- Soy lecithin
- Soy milk
- Soybean oil
- Spinach
- Strawberries
- Sweet potatoes
- Tempeh
- Tofu
- Turnips

Another time I had a negative effect from a goitrogenic food is when I decided to make myself some miso soup with organic miso (soy), after not having any soy or miso for years. The organic soy didn't matter because within 30 minutes of eating a bowl of miso soup, my thyroid swelled and started to itch. My entire body and extremities became freezing cold as my thyroid was suppressed. My lungs also felt full and it was getting hard to breathe. I mistakenly went to the emergency room and waited for hours only to find that the doctors couldn't offer any help. After I arrived home from the emergency room, I immediately started taking about 4 Tablespoons of coconut oil per day, used spirulina to detox the soy and only ate foods that fed the thyroid. Again, those of us diagnosed with low thyroid will need to be careful with the goitrogenic foods the rest of our lives. It took about 2 days for my body temperature to return to normal and for my thyroid to stop itching.

If you are going to enlist only the juice fast as opposed to vegetable smoothies, you can also use some psyllium husk or fresh ground flax seeds to get your fiber to help eliminate the constipation, see the colon cleansing chapter for that information. A juice fast is a great cleanse for some people but it may not be beneficial to another depending upon your current state of health. Contact a qualified naturopathic or integrative doctor and ask them if this type of cleanse will benefit you. Another way to detoxify the body, which is written about in biblical texts, is the water fast.

13

Water Fasting

What happens when you have tried every method of detoxification and nothing seems to be working for you? This is when your health and detoxification needs to be taken to the next level and embark upon the most extreme detox regimen of all; The Water Fast.

According to the Book "The Miracle of Fasting," Fasting can aid in the elimination process, restores strength and vitality, often relieves tension and insomnia, slows the ageing process, can eliminate addictions, eliminates deadly acid crystals within the body and joints, cleanses mucous toxins, eliminates body odors, promotes healthy elimination, and more. (1).

There are occasions when all of the previous detoxification methods will not work for various issues. The main reason may be due to a biofilm, systemic candida condition and/or parasitic infestation in the digestive tract, which are several of the most difficult conditions to rid from the body. There are also certain autoimmune conditions where the water fast is the only method that may work to re-set the body.

Before I had learned of biofilms in my body, I had turned to water fasting because the systemic candida within my bloodstream and leaky gut had caused so many problems that none of the other detoxification methods were working any longer, when they previously worked before. I therefore, turned to water fasting and continued coffee enemas to cleanse the liver of increased toxins being released through fasting.

One of the benefits of water fasting is that it gives your digestive tract a much needed rest so it is able to repair itself. The digestive tract normally takes 14 days to heal completely, so if you have extreme intestinal permeability issues, this can help you to heal. Although, for those with severe leaky gut (intestinal permeability), it will take much longer than 14 days to heal the gut lining. I can speak from personal experience that it can take years to successfully heal the body of chronic conditions; such as, leaky gut, irritable bowel disease, small intestinal bacterial overgrowth (SIBO), severe adrenal fatigue, systemic candida, autoimmune conditions, etc.

What I noticed through water fasting is that if you have systemic candida in the digestive tract, you will notice that your tongue becomes white as the candida is leaving the body, increased body odors, pasty mouth, bad breath, acne, rashes, and boils will come out, and you may experience many of the other healing crisis symptoms discussed in the next section. You will also notice lots of mucous, slime and parasites may be expelled during water fasting.

The first three days of the water fast are the most difficult as you are releasing many toxins and may experience extreme fatigue, headaches and other symptoms of the healing crisis. Although, you aren't eating any food you do not experience hunger for quite a while. Every time you have a hunger pang is usually a cry for thirst, so it is best to drink some water at that time. True hunger will return in time. You will lose a lot of weight on this fast at the rate of about 1-2 lbs. per day. Keep in mind that after you break the fast, you will gain about 10 lbs. of that lost weight back. But with the majority of toxins released from your body, the weight should stay off as long as you don't go back to your old eating habits of processed foods and sugars.

To break the fast, you have to go very slow with very juicy fruits and broths at first to replace lost metabolites. I like eating lots of watermelon, bone broth, or chicken broth in the first days after breaking the fast, and then I may add in some avocado. Think of soft foods that are easy to digest are the best to start off with when you break your fast. You will not be able to eat as much as before you fasted, so a few chunks of watermelon may fill you for a meal. I always start the first day after a fast with just watermelon, broth, and some coconut water. The next day I will add in the avocado to the watermelon and coconut water. The third day after breaking the fast, I may add in some scrambled eggs.

Those who should not undertake lengthy water fasts are those with severe chronic conditions where your immune system has been compromised for a long period of time. The reason is that this can cause your adrenal glands to fail because they aren't being nourished properly with ingesting only water. This happened to me when I had done a few water fasts in 2013 and 2014 to heal the severe leaky gut and SIBO, but finally was diagnosed with severe adrenal fatigue in October of 2014. My immune system was not strong enough to sustain lengthy water fasting and my adrenal glands suffered the consequences.

Water fasting is biblical and has been done for thousands of years. Although, water fasting should be monitored closely by a qualified physician to monitor blood pressure, heart rate, and pulse. There is even specific water fasting retreats where you can complete a water fasting program safely and be monitored the entire time. For those who want to go to a retreat for water fasting, I suggest Tanglewood Wellness Center, run by Loren Lockwood and located in Costa Rica. Their website is www.tanglewoodwellnesscenter.com.

I do not suggest starting off with the lengthy water fast because it is so extreme and needs to be monitored. However, when all other avenues of detoxification have been exhausted unsuccessfully, water fasting may be an option for you. Please discuss this with your qualified naturopathic doctor or go to the water fasting retreat listed above.

There are certain conditions when water fasting is not a good idea; such as, those who are chronically ill with compromised immune systems due to late stage cancer and other diseases, extended water fasting of longer than 2-3 days can cause a metabolic disorder and cause your adrenal glands to crash causing adrenal fatigue. I do not recommend extended water fasts of longer than a couple of days at a time without the supervision of a qualified, knowledgeable practitioner to monitor you. The reason I have concern about the water fast is that I had done quite a few water fasts in 2013, with the longest being 33 days. It did help to heal my leaky gut a bit and healed the SIBO infection in my gut, but it also compromised my adrenal glands and I was later diagnosed with severe stage 3C adrenal fatigue in October of 2014 of which I also ended up healing naturally.

Intermittent Water Fasting:

Intermittent fasting of a few hours to days at a time can help tremendously to get rid of inflammation and illness. However, if you are chronically ill with a compromised immune system currently, lengthy water fasting may be too drastic for your body to handle at this time and you should stick to 24 hours at a time until your body is stronger and you have detoxed much of the toxins.

After I had been healing my adrenal glands for over a year and a half, I embarked on a one-day water fast, once a week. This is where you abstain from all food and just drink pure water for the day whenever you are thirsty or have hunger pangs. At the end of the twenty-four hours at my next bowel movement I would notice a release of a lot of yeast and some parasites. Even though you can eat perfectly healthy with no GMOs, No gluten, No dairy, and all vegetables, parasites and candida can still grow within the intestines and sometimes the water fast is very beneficial in cleansing the system.

According to Dr. Paul and Dr. Patricia Bragg in their book, "The Miracle of Fasting," "fasting will not only purify the body and help to restore it to well-being, but has a great effect on the mental and spiritual parts of man." (1). For those new to water fasting, you should only start out with a 24 - 36 hour fast once a week because shorter fasts are safer and don't require medical supervision. The reason they are safer is that if you do a longer fast too begin with, you are dumping too many toxins into the body and it can be harmful especially for those who are chronically ill. Shorter fasts can help to eliminate the toxins at a slower pace and you can still experience healing in the long run. Once your body is comfortable with the 24-36 hour fast and your body has eliminated many of the toxins, you would be able to undertake a longer fast, such as 3-4 days or 7-10 days.

Just as it is important to learn how to fast properly, it is also important to know how to break a fast properly. When breaking a fast, do not overeat, eat some watermelon, lightly steamed greens, avocado or another vegetable or fruit that is easily digestible. I generally like breaking a fast with soup broth, bone broth, watermelon, avocado or steamed greens; nothing too heavy. As the days' pass, I would add in scrambled eggs as my appetite begins to return.

Bible References for Fasting:

Ezra 8: 22-23: "…….our God protects all those who worship him, but his fierce anger rages against those who abandon him. So we fasted and earnestly prayed that our God would take care of us, and he heard our prayer." (NLT).

Joel 1:14: Announce a time of fasting; call the people together for a solemn meeting. Bring the leaders and all the people into the Temple of the Lord your God, and cry out to him there. (NLT).

Matthew 6:16-18: And when you fast, don't make it obvious, as the hypocrites do, who try to look pale and disheveled so people will admire them for their fasting. I assure you, that is the only reward they will ever get. But when you fast, comb your hair and wash your face. Then no one will suspect you are fasting, except your Father, who knows what you do in secret. And your Father, who knows all secrets, will reward you. (NLT).

Matthew 9: 14-17: One day the disciples of John the Baptist came to Jesus and asked him, "Why do we and the Pharisees fast, but your disciples don't fast?" Jesus responded "Should the wedding guests mourn while celebrating with the groom? Someday he will be taken from them, and then they will fast. And who would patch an old garment with unshrunk cloth? For the patch shrinks and pulls away from the old cloth, leaving an even bigger hole than before. And no one puts new wine into old wineskins. The old skins would burst from the pressure, spilling the wine and ruining the skins. New wine must be stored in new wineskins. That way both the wine and the wineskin are preserved." (NLT).

My personal preference is the intermittent water fast, and I have done both. The reason is that is not as hard on the body, you can always work your way up to a lengthier water fast when your body has dumped much of the toxins in the intermittent fasting period and you are stronger. With any type of fast, you need to make sure that your body is strong enough to sustain a fast and be beneficial for you. If you are suffering from adrenal issues, any type of water fast (lengthy or intermittent) may not be beneficial for you and can make you worse. Listen to your body and consult a qualified physician for guidance.

14

Additional Detox Methods

The additional detox methods are beneficial to complete at the same time of completing any and all of the other detoxes in this book. Meaning that you still need to detoxify the inside of your body, but these additional detoxification methods will also help to facilitate healing the body in conjunction with the traditional detoxification methods mentioned in the book.

Oil Pulling:

Oil pulling is an ancient practice of swishing oil around in your mouth and through your teeth. The health benefits of oil pulling are tightening of gums, whitening of teeth, detoxing the upper respiratory tract, keeping plaque at bay, and fresher breath.

I have personally been practicing oil pulling since 2007 and have tried every type of oil on the market. I have found that unrefined sesame oil works the best for oil pulling and I have gotten the best results with this type of oil. I will also use virgin coconut oil when I run out of the unrefined sesame oil. Oil pulling has whitened my teeth naturally, even though I smoked for 23 years. It has also tightened my gums around some loose teeth that I had, which prevented me from needing to remove those teeth for many years. Whenever I go to a dentist, they are amazed at how good my teeth look despite the major dental problems I have. I do have advanced periodontal disease and the dentists kept threatening that my teeth would fall out of my mouth any day now, they have been saying that since 2007.

To begin oil pulling; put a teaspoon full of unrefined sesame oil (I use spectrum brand) into your mouth and begin swishing the oil back and forth through your teeth. It feels weird at first and you only may be able to do this for a few minutes at a time and work your way up to 20 minutes per day. DO NOT swallow the oil; as the oil in your mouth is picking up and "pulling" toxins from the mouth and upper respiratory tract and that oil will contain toxins. After swishing the oil for 20 minutes, spit the oil into the trash and rinse out your mouth with clean water. You can then brush your teeth. I like to do this practice first thing when I wake up in the morning before eating or drinking anything. I usually do the oil pulling while I am feeding my cats and getting my breakfast ready.

Dry Skin Brushing:

Start with a good, stiff skin brush. My favorite is the Yerba Prima brand skin brush. When you brush your skin, you experience softer skin by sloughing off the dead layer of cells. You are also stimulating your lymph by dry skin brushing as well. There were many times when I had hard lumps show up underneath my armpits, in my lymph nodes from detoxing, and after a few times of dry skin brushing, the toxic lumps dissipated.

To dry skin brush, start with brushing your back and buttocks. Then, to do the front, start from the tops of your feet and move up your legs. Always brush in an upward motion. Move to the trunk of your body and chest area. Brush your hands and up your arms to underneath your armpits. Always brush toward your heart. Once you have brushed your entire body, you can take a shower to remove the dead skin cells and toxins from your body. You will notice that your skin will become much softer over time, where you don't need lotion and if you shave, your shaves will be much smoother as well because you brushed the hairs away from the follicle, to make for a nice, smooth shave.

Dry Heat Saunas:

Sweating is key to detoxing because the skin is our largest organ and when you are detoxing, many poisons will come out of your skin in the form of rashes, acne, boils, cysts, etc. By utilizing a dry heat sauna, you are causing your body to sweat out the toxins quicker. Plus, being in a dry heat sauna just feels great on the body. Make sure to shower after the sauna to wash off all the toxins which came out of your body.

Exercise:

Exercise is imperative to healing naturally and it also makes you sweat, which is a great detox mechanism. Exercise can be in whatever form you enjoy. I personally hate going to a gym, so I opt for hiking in nature, ice skating, cross country skiing, snow shoeing, or any outdoor activities. Do something you enjoy for exercise and that will help you to keep with the regimen.

I started hiking in 2009, when I had cancer, which was also when I quit smoking. Exercise was a great way to get my mind away from smoking, so every time I thought of smoking, I went hiking instead. The exercise is great to get rid of those toxins in your body. Plus, the exercise can help to boost your serotonin levels, which will boost your mood.

Rebounding:

Rebounding involves jumping on a mini trampoline or any kind of trampoline, to stimulate the lymph nodes in your body and keep them healthy by removing toxins from clogged lymph nodes. Mini trampolines are sold many places for a reasonable price, so everyone can get into the habit of rebounding for a few minutes per day.

Eventually, you will want to work your way up to 20 minutes a day of rebounding, but starting out with a few minutes at a time is fine. Do what you can at first and don't be too hard on yourself if you can only do 30 seconds, you will notice over time that you will get better and feel better.

Activated Charcoal:

Activated charcoal is sold in capsule form in health food stores and online. It is used to detoxify poisons from the body, so it is helpful for food poisoning, alcohol poisoning, drug overdose, traveler's diarrhea, poisonous insect bites, bacterial infections, and tooth infections.

Activated Charcoal capsules are a "must-have" in every household. Activated Charcoal is a binding agent which attracts toxins and carries them out of the body. You can take activated charcoal internally for food poisoning, alcohol toxicity, or even to prevent hangovers. You can also make activated charcoal into a paste and use it externally for tooth aches, insect bites, spider bites, gum infections, etc.

I have personally used activated charcoal for both internal and external factors. I have successfully used it a few times for gum and tooth infections, where I made the activated charcoal into a thick paste and wrapped the charcoal paste in cheesecloth and slept with it on the gum infection overnight. Within a few nights, the gum infection is cleared, the pain is gone, and I saved myself an expensive trip to the dentist. I also open up the capsules and mix the activated charcoal into my weekly face mask to clear up any acne, eczema, or psoriasis.

To make a paste out of activated charcoal; empty approximately 6 capsules of activated charcoal into a small bowl and add 1-2 drops of unrefined sesame oil or virgin coconut oil. Stir the activated charcoal and oil to make a thick paste, you may need to add more oil, but not too much, as it needs to be a thick paste. The paste should be thick enough to form a firm ball. Then you can place the paste on any wound, infection, or insect bite to soak up the toxins and cover the paste with a band-aid or gauze. For gum and tooth infections, place the charcoal paste into a square of cheesecloth and tuck it into the gum line where the infection is located and sleep with it overnight daily until the infection is cleared. Make sure to make a fresh charcoal paste nightly if you are using it for infections. You can also use activated charcoal to whiten your teeth by brushing with the charcoal powder, although this is very messy and it does take a while to get the black grit out of your teeth afterward.

Activated charcoal also works wonders for internal toxicity. I have personally used activated charcoal whenever I had food poisoning or was planning on having a few drinks at a party. For food poisoning, I take 2 capsules and wait to see if it is working or not before I take more. For alcohol, I take 1 capsule per alcoholic beverage. Be aware that activated charcoal taken internally can cause constipation for a couple of days so make sure you take it for a very good reason and drink plenty of water to stay hydrated. The activated charcoal will also make your stool black, so don't be weary if you see black stool the first time you have a bowel movement after taking activated charcoal capsules. You may even notice yeast or parasites attached to your stool the next time you have a bowel movement as activated charcoal does bind to toxins.

Activated charcoal capsules can be found at any health food store, vitamin store or online and should be a staple in every household. You should also make a habit of carrying this miracle pill with you on trips as a precaution in case of food, poisoning, water poisoning, or bug bites.

Emotional Detox:

What happens when you have tried to detoxify your body, you changed your diet, you have gotten rid of the root causes (infections), but you still are not seeing any results? It is time to look toward changing your mind set and attitude. I know how hard it is to be chronically ill for a long period of time, I know how difficult it is to cry yourself to sleep because you are just so exhausted from being sick and tired all the time, I know how exhausting it is to heal your body naturally and go through the detoxes time and time again, and I know what it is like to feel complete loneliness and despair from not having anyone who understands because most people are brainwashed into believing that western medicine is the only way and falsely believe doctors are God.

I also know what it is like to have people be rude and mean to you for no reason other than they are just hateful, jealous peoples. I have seen my share of horrible people who will attack those who are sick and healing their bodies naturally, it is shocking really. It is difficult not to get bitter and blame God, but that is the last thing you should do and I know how hard that is to do. The best way to heal your emotions and detox your life is too forgive. You must forgive those people who have harmed you. I am not saying that you need to hang around those toxic people because that is not beneficial to your life or health, but you can forgive them and move on, just to help yourself. By not forgiving them, you are only hurting yourself because those toxic emotions will keep you sick.

Stop being angry at God. Like the story of Job; God may have allowed Satan to attack you with sickness, but ask yourself why? God must be preparing you for something great and he is testing your character and faith in him. Every time I would get sick with yet another chronic illness, I would ask God why and I realized that Satan kept attacking me because God must have a great plan for my life. If this sounds all too familiar, keep rebuking Satan and keep asking God to bind Satan's hands from doing any more harm in your life.

Two of my favorite verses from Isaiah that I repeated to myself multiple times daily during my eight long years of cancer and chronic illness are that "No Weapon formed against me shall ever prosper" and "The Lord will be my vindicator." The exact verse is found in Isaiah 54:17, "No weapon that is formed against you will prosper; and every tongue that accuses you in judgment you will condemn. This is the heritage of the servants of the LORD, and their vindication is from Me," declares the LORD. (New American Standard Bible). The more I repeated this verse; I saw things begin to happen. I was vindicated against many of those people who lied against me and were unkind.

It really helps with emotional detox to go somewhere where you feel safe, happy, and peaceful, where you can reach out to God. For me, hiking in the mountains is where I feel happiest and closest to God. I always pray while I am hiking, mainly to thank God for his advanced healing. I also feel so much closer to God when I am in his mountains amongst the beauty of the forest and breathing in the fresh air. I think that every breath I take is one step closer to being healthy again. Think of all of the beautiful places on earth that God created that you can enjoy, some of you may also feel closer to God while you are in church enjoying fellowship with fellow believers. The point is to go where you feel closest to God and talk to him, he will listen.

Positive thinking is another key to healing. Listen to positive messages daily in any form that makes you happy. Do activities that make you happy because happiness is crucial to creating lasting health and wellness. Think positive, happy thoughts, and they will come to fruition. You must remain positive if you expect to heal, as the words you speak are powerful and will come true. So, if you speak words of death, then that is what will happen. Speak words of life and living and give those words life with your actions. You can't just sit around and wait for someone to do the work for you; God wants to see how badly you want to live by the active role you will take in your own healing.

To Sum up the Emotional Detox:

1. **Pray:** pray daily or hourly if needed.

2. **Forgive:** forgive those who have harmed you and move on.

3. **Think** Positive, Happy thoughts

4. **"Feel"** that you are already healed and keep repeating it to yourself daily or hourly if needed.

15

Detoxification Symptoms

Many people will start a detox regimen to heal their ailments, yet stop the detoxification process midstream because they begin to feel horrible. They feel like they are getting worse and so they may become doubtful and stop detoxifying their bodies. The truth is that your body is expelling toxins associated with disease, which is what is causing you to feel horrible in the beginning phases of a detox. This experience is referred to as a Herxheimer reaction and is normal in the course of detoxification.

The Herxheimer reaction originated from two dermatologists working with patients. "The phenomenon was first described by Adolf Jarisch (1860-1902) working in Vienna, Austria, and a few years later by Karl Herxheimer (1861-1942), working in Frankfort, Germany. Both doctors were dermatologists, mainly treating syphilitic lesions of the skin. They noticed that in response to treatment, many patients developed not only fever, perspiration, night sweats, nausea and vomiting, but their skin lesions became larger and more inflamed before
settling down and healing. Interestingly, they found that those who had the most extreme reactions healed the best and fastest. The patient might be ill for 2-3 days, but then their lesions resolved." (1).

Herxheimer reactions can occur as the body adjusts to the die-off process and responds to the increased load on the lymphatic system, particularly in cases of systemic and chronic conditions and/or severe infections. The term Herxheimer reaction is more commonly called a "Healing Crisis," which is much easier to pronounce.

The major elimination channels are the colon, urethra, the mouth, nasal passages, and the skin. These are the areas in which you may notice a healing crisis happening. While detoxifying the body, you will most likely experience flu like symptoms that may last a few days or more. This is a sign that your body is ridding itself of toxins. Any ailments you have had in the past will come out in reverse order of when you first experienced them. These symptoms tell you that the detoxification process is working. Here are some other die-off symptoms which you may experience.

- Headache, fatigue, dizziness, nausea, diarrhea, bloating, gas, constipation, excess gas, and burping.
- Increased joint or muscle pain, swollen glands, elevated heart   rate, sweating, and fever.
- Chills, cold feeling in your extremities, recurring vaginal, prostate, and sinus infections.
- Body itchiness, hives, skin breakouts, acne, boils, or rashes.

If the "healing crisis" is too severe, you may want to slow down a bit, so as not to release too many toxins at once. To slow down the detox process, you can reduce the dosage of whichever cleanse you are conducting. You can also help to release the toxins quicker by drinking more water, using dry heat saunas, infrared saunas, exercise, rest, coffee enemas, and take 2,000 mg of vitamin C daily.

By conducting these cleanses, you will be able to free yourself from the many ailments that may have plagued you for years. Keep on a regular plan to detoxify your body at least annually. Those with cancer or other chronic conditions should detoxify their bodies twice a year at least. I like to detox as the New Year begins, but it can be done at any time you feel sluggish or need a boost.

All the methods of detoxifying the body will help to rid your body of toxins, try the different cleanses and see which ones work best for you. Do not perform them all at the same time or you could detoxify your body too fast, which will cause further health problems. Go slow, relax, and know that you are doing a great thing for your body and helping to prevent disease or rid your body of disease.

When detoxing from cancer, especially advanced cancer, you may experience what is known as Lysing symptoms. In layman's terms, Lysing is just the breaking down of the cancer cell, which releases additional potassium, uric acid, and phosphorous into the blood. Lysing also depletes calcium reserves. If after starting any alternative treatments or detox regimen; you experience extreme headaches, vomiting, diarrhea, muscle cramps, lethargy, or confusion, this means that the toxins from the cancer or other diseases are being released too quickly. Coffee enemas can help to alleviate pain and flush the toxins from the liver. Liquid bentonite clay, activated charcoal, spirulina, dandelion, milk thistle, and N-acetyl cysteine (NAC) are a few methods that help to bind toxins and flush them out of the body.

Lysing symptoms that go on for an extended period can lead to kidney failure, cardiovascular issues, seizures, and other organ damage due to the amount of toxins being dumped into the liver, which may re-intoxicate the body. It is important that if you experience lysing symptoms, to spread out your alternative treatments, utilize coffee enemas, and liquid bentonite clay and/or activated charcoal to alleviate the toxic load on the body.

When I was detoxing from cancer, I experienced lysing in the form of a rash around my neck. Cancer can show itself in many forms when it is detoxing from your body. The rash had shown up a few months after I had begun the various alternative cancer protocols and eventually lasted seven months before my body was detoxed from the cancer and that is when the rash had finally dissipated. This rash was confirmed as an epidermal growth factor receptor rash, which is indicative of cancer being within the body. You cannot possibly have the epidermal growth factor receptor rash if you do not first have cancer.

The Epidermal Growth Factor Receptor (EGFR) is, "The protein found on the surface of some cells and to which epidermal growth factor binds, causing the cells to divide. It is found at abnormally high levels on the surface of many types of cancer cells, so these cells may divide excessively in the presence of epidermal growth factor." The EGFR is locked within the protein of the cancer cell and when released, it can appear in the form of a rash. In layman's terms, it is when there is an increased layer of protein covering the cancer cell and is more prevalent in the advanced stages (stage 3 or 4) of HER1 types of cancer. Those with HER1 type advanced cancers that may experience the EGFR rash are those people with non-small cell lung cancer, breast cancer, pancreatic cancer, ovarian cancer, head and neck cancers. Those cancer patients that experienced the EGFR type rash had a better survival rate than those that hadn't experienced the EGFR with a HER1 type cancer. The presence of a rash in these types of cancers is a good sign that cancer is leaving your body. You can roughly determine your stage of cancer by the length of time you have the EGFR rash.

While I was detoxing my body from cancer; the nutritionist, biochemist, and other cancer survivors I had spoken with had confirmed that the presence of a rash on the upper chest or neck is a sign that either breast cancer or non-small cell lung cancer is detoxing from the body. I needed to consult with these individuals because I was starting to worry as to why the rash had not went away as of yet. I was informed that the rash would not subside until my body was cleared of all cancer and the rash could last a very long time depending upon the severity and stage of cancer that I had. I had spoken to a woman; who was diagnosed stage 4 breast cancer, who had told me that her rash had lasted just short of a year. I had also spoken to my mother, who had stage 3 breast cancer, and she said that her lymph nodes were barely swollen and didn't ache like mine. My mother also never experienced a rash, although she opted for an integrative approach, which may have interfered with the natural healing process. Considering that my rash didn't dissipate for seven months and my lymph nodes were visibly swollen and constantly in pain, would put me at a pretty serious stage of cancer.

Even when you are detoxing from other chronic illness, that isn't cancer, you may experience some pretty harsh detox symptoms. I have experienced everything from rashes, to cysts on my back and face, lots of yeast and/or parasites coming out of stool, brain fog or cloudy thinking, dyslexic symptoms, vomiting, diarrhea, constipation, ear aches, teeth throbbing, pain in joints, thick mucus coming out of my nose, white/patchy tongue, and more. None of these are pleasant symptoms, but they are signs that your detox regimen is working.

When you are detoxing, your ailments will come out in the reverse order of when you first had that disease or ailment. For instance, if you had acne when you were young and had asthma when you were older, you will begin to detoxify the body of the asthma symptoms before you detoxify your body from the acne symptoms. You will also experience a lesser version of the original ailment as it detoxes from your body.

An example from my own experience is when I had the EGFR rash around my neck in 2009-2010 and then many chronic illnesses after that. While I was detoxing, I had experienced the EGFR rash again, which appeared in a lesser form, as it detoxed from my cells. Each time I detoxify my body, another layer comes from my cells to renew itself and I experience a new healing crisis that comes out of my body because I am going a layer deeper.

The primary organ, which helps to rid the body of toxins, is the liver. The liver works primarily to flush toxins from the body. However, when your body has too many toxins coursing through the liver at one time, the liver can be overburdened and you can re-intoxicate yourself because the toxins will get re-circulated back into the body instead of being released by the liver. It is important to make sure to detoxify your body slowly so your liver can do its job. If you have too many symptoms of a healing crisis and feel really bad, you can always do a coffee enema to release the toxins from the liver. This will help you to feel better quickly and help the liver do its job.

Think of it like this; have you ever been out for a night of partying and you have a hangover the next day due to alcohol poisoning? The pain of the hangover is your body's way of ridding your body of the toxic effects of the alcohol; you have a headache because your liver is overworking itself by trying to process the alcohol out of your system. When the body is finally clear of the alcoholic toxins bombarding your liver, you will feel better. The same is true of any toxin in the body. The toxins are trying to get out and the skin is the largest organ, therefore you may experience boils, cysts, body odor and rashes coming out of your pores because your liver is overburdened with carting the toxins out of the body.

If you do experience a healing crisis, know that your body is healing and the healing crisis will not last forever. You will feel much better once the healing crisis passes and you are free from disease. Now that you know how to detoxify the body and the healing crisis you may experience, you can move on to what to feed the body to reverse multiple diseases naturally. In the following chapters, I will be discussing the various diets to heal your body naturally.

16

Which Cleanses Work Best?

I am always asked which detox kits to use or which ones work the best. Which detoxification regimens work best depends upon your individual level of toxicity and the level of illness within your own body. I have met people who swear by certain supplements or detoxes but when I tried them, they never worked the same for me. The reason is that I was dealing with severe leaky gut, SIBO, biofilms, and other issues in which I would absorb no supplements in pill form whatsoever, so all the detoxes were lost on me. Eventually, I had to resort to everything in powder or liquid form and healing the gut lining before my body began to detoxify itself properly.

Some people will be able to pick up a detox kit at the local health food store and that may be enough for them. However, there are many of you who will need a more thorough detox to reach multiple layers of toxins that are trapped within your cells, which may have caused extreme inflammation and chronic disease. For those who are chronically ill, you will have to detoxify the body slowly, layer by layer, and this can take years to finally get to the very root cause of your disease and heal completely through detoxification.

Using the detoxes in order of the colon, candida, parasite, kidney and liver allows you to go slower, at your own pace and focus on that one area/problem at one time for a specific length of time. Some people may only need a few days of the colon detox, while others may need an entire week or two. For the candida cleanse, if you are chronically ill, chances are good that candida is one of the root causes of your health issue and you may need to repeat this specific cleanse for years, along with the anti-candida diet until you improve. The same is true with the parasite cleanse as it may need repeating, depending upon whether or not you have parasites and how infected with parasites you are. The kidney cleanse and liver cleanse can also be repeated until you are experiencing increased wellness. If you find that after all of the detoxes that your body is still sick, you may need to look at deeper root causes; such as, viral infections, bacterial infections, parasitic infections, fungal infections, and biofilms.

As you begin to get well, you can try out other detoxes; such as the intermittent fasting or the juice fasting cleanse. These are a bit more advanced because you are skipping meals, giving your digestion a rest and therefore, will be dumping a lot of toxins all at once. For those who are not too toxic to begin with, it may be manageable to conduct a water or juice fast as your main detox regimen. For others with chronic conditions, you may need to slowly get rid of the layers of toxins before advancing to a more strenuous water or juice fast.

The key is to be patient and listen to your body, which is easier said than done, because it can literally take years of continued detoxing and change of diet to finally get better. What you must realize is that every single time you detoxify your body, you are removing one more layer of toxins and you are one day closer to being completely well.

Many people ask me what they should eat while they are detoxing their bodies or how to continue to feel well after their detoxes. Complete healing and longevity is all about the foods you eat. Face it, if you were eating healthy to begin with, you may not have ended up with chronic illness. So, it is imperative to change your diet during your detox and continue on the path to wellness by adopting a new lifestyle of eating healthier. I'm not saying that you can't cheat once in a while because none of us are perfect, but stick to a clean diet as best as possible in order to experience and maintain wellness.

17

What Should I Eat?

There are so many books, websites, doctors, and nutritionists out there telling people which diet is best. The mass of information on special diets is confusing because most of this information is written by people who have never truly been sick and they don't speak from personal experience. When someone has never been truly sick, any diet would work well because their body is still working at optimum performance. The problem lies when you are chronically ill and your body is no longer working properly or responding, then what?

So, which diet works best to heal the body when you have disease and want to detoxify the body? The answer to that question is dependent upon the type of disease you are trying to reverse, the level of toxicity in the body, if you have biofilm infections, diets you have undertaken previously, whether you have done chemotherapy or radiation, supplement use, antibiotic usage, and how the specific diet plan makes you feel.

I also choose to not call it a diet, but it needs to be lifestyle changes to not only become healthier, but to stay that way. If you change your diet and get healthy but then go back to eating the trashy way you used too, your body will only get sick again. Does this mean that you will never be able to eat the foods you enjoy again? No, you can cheat occasionally after you are well, just don't make a habit of it and make sure to continue to detoxify your body at least once a year to get rid of the toxins you ingested.

Cancer and other diseases can be caused from eating meat and dairy, which contain hormones, antibiotics, and steroids. The pancreatic enzymes in your body cannot digest meat products as easily as vegetables. The digestive system becomes blocked and works less efficiently over time. Such foods need to be completely avoided while undertaking a diet to reverse cancer.

The reason to avoid meat and dairy, while you are healing cancer or some other chronic diseases, is because you need the pancreatic enzymes to break down the protein coating surrounding the cancer cell wall and not the protein from meat, ice cream, cheese and eggs from non-organic sources. Pancreatic or proteolytic enzymes need to be available to break down the protein barrier of the cancer cell instead of working on digesting the meat from your last meal. These enzymes are instrumental in oxygenating the cancer cells and helping to reverse them back to normal cells.

When I was healing cancer, I stayed away from meats for a year to ensure that the pancreatic enzymes, in the form of pineapple, I was ingesting were working to break down my cancer cells, and not working on breaking down my meal. I would cheat occasionally on Thanksgiving and Christmas with organic Turkey or have some wild fish and eggs sparingly.

Many cancer patients, especially if they are in the advanced stages, may have issues with their digestive system and may have what is known as intestinal permeability. This is where your digestive system is impaired by holes within the small intestines, as I discussed in the section on leaky gut. As I was healing severe leaky gut, food allergies, SIBO and asthma, I had to steer clear of dairy, gluten, soy, sugars, all processed foods, hormone laden meats, caffeine, alcohol, and GMOs. All of these foods would cause me extreme distress with allergic reactions happening 10 minutes after I had eaten any of the offending foods. At first, I didn't notice the symptoms because they didn't happen too often. It became very clear later when it leads to my suffering with extreme irritable bowel syndrome for an entire year. I also wasn't absorbing any nutrients that I was ingesting and this became a problem in trying to heal my body. I literally could not eat any vegetables or any raw foods because I could not digest most foods.

This is what is so frustrating for those of us who have been chronically ill. There is a plethora of health websites, articles, and books that are written by people who have never been sick who tell you that you should just eat their way and you will be healed, but that isn't the entire truth because there are so many other factors involved.

During this process of trying different dietary plans, I had realized that not everyone can eat vegan, vegetarian, or raw successfully because we all have different body chemistry. In addition to that, many of us may be in various stages of cancer, chronic illness, or intestinal permeability that minimize the organs' ability to digest raw vegetables properly. You have to find which foods work well with your body type to reap the greatest benefits.

While I was healing adrenal fatigue, I had to enlist a completely different dietary change, then when I had cancer, because my body required different foods and nutrients to be able to heal. I had to introduce more pink salt to feed the adrenals, salt everything, and I ate more potatoes and proteins to heal. I still could not process raw foods at this stage.

I have tried every dietary change out there from paleo, auto-immune protocol, allergen free, GAPS diet, vegan, vegetarian, FODMAP friendly, ketogenic and so on. I have narrowed it down to the best dietary guidelines out there where you can choose which one may be the right one for you. If one dietary principle doesn't work well for you, switch to something else, as this is not a one-size, fits-all approach.

I know that changing the way you eat is difficult, especially if you have a family who is not on board with you. It was easier for me because I had nobody to cook for, so I could easily change my eating habits without backlash from anyone mostly. For those of you with families, you can ask your family to get on board this healthy change with you or they will just have to understand that you being healthy is the most important thing and that your dietary changes are a necessary part of your healing process. Possibly it may inspire them in time to want to change with you. After all, how can you possibly take care of anyone else if you don't take care of yourself first? This change has to be about you and regaining your health.

I have embraced a new way of eating over the past eight years which is healthier and have adopted it as a lifestyle change, which I will explain in a later chapter. The word "diet" alludes to a temporary situation, therefore, you must embrace a "lifestyle change" or "dietary change" to make a lasting improvement in your everyday plan.

18

The Paleo Diet

The Paleo diet consists of eating the way our ancestors ate. This theory is based upon the Paleolithic period and cavemen who didn't have processed foods, salt, etc. So, this diet is based upon eating high protein, lots of vegetables, nuts and fruits. No dairy, no bread, no processed foods, and no salt are allowed, as they say that the ancestors never had any of these items.

Another alteration of this method of eating is also called the Autoimmune Protocol Diet (AIP); which is another form of the Paleo diet except you cut out all trigger foods that cause auto-immune illness; such as, gluten, dairy, eggs, soy, nuts, nightshades, histamine foods, etc.

To simplify this diet, you can eat all the lean meats, fish, and seafood you can eat. All fruits and non-starchy vegetables are also legal to eat. You are not allowed any cereals, legumes, dairy products, or processed foods. You may eat healthy, good fats; such as, avocados, avocado oil, coconut oil, omega 3 fats like flaxseed oil, fish oil, and olive oil.

According to Loren Cordain, who wrote the book on the Paleo Diet, he says that there are seven keys to the Paleo diet; which are:

- Eat a high amount of animal protein.
- Eat fewer carbohydrates, from fruits and vegetables only. No grains, potatoes or refined sugars.
- Eat lots of fiber from non-starchy fruits and vegetables.
- Eat a moderate amount of good fats and equal amounts of omega 3 to omega 6 fats.
- Eat foods high in potassium, but low in sodium content.
- Eat a diet which is pH balanced to support bone health.
- Eat foods rich in plant phytochemicals, vitamins, minerals, and antioxidants.

Whether or not this lifestyle dietary change will work for you really depends upon your current state of health. This is a low carb diet and I am no longer a big fan of low carb dieting; although it may work for you in the beginning, it can further harm those who are chronically ill. Low carb dieting over time can alter hormonal function, especially in women, causing further problems.

Again, you may need to work with a qualified nutritionist to guide you based upon your current state of health and what will work for your body to ensure the best results.

19

The GAPS Diet

Natasha Campbell McBride founded the Gut and Psychology Syndrome diet (known as the GAPS diet), which uses bone broth and fermented foods to heal the gut lining; which can aid in healing diseases such as autism, ADD, ADHD, leaky gut, depression, schizophrenia, etc. I have used this diet to help heal my gut lining and still use bone broth to this day, but it did take a lot more than just bone broth to help heal the severity of my leaky gut condition. This diet is for very severe health conditions and you may be undertaking this diet for years to heal properly and completely. Along with detoxification, this diet can help the body to heal from disease naturally.

Three Phases of the GAPS Diet:

1. Intro GAPS diet

2. Second phase

3. Reintroduction of foods phase

STAGE 1:

The Stage 1 of the GAPS diet consists of homemade meat stock (beef, lamb, bison, chicken, turkey, pheasant or fish), soups or stews with well cooked vegetables, probiotic fermented foods, fresh chamomile, ginger or herbal teas, and purified water.

When I first began on the GAPS protocol, I could not tolerate any vegetables (raw or cooked), nor could I tolerate high histamine foods; such as sauerkraut or other fermented foods. So, all that left me with in the beginning was to drink bone broth and drink herbal teas. I was on this stage for quite a while before

I was well enough to begin to add meats into the bone broth and then it took a bit longer before I was able to add vegetables into the broth. It literally took years before I could tolerate any fermented foods, although I still have some trouble with high histamine foods.

STAGE 2:

In stage 2, you can continue with Stage 1 foods. It is important to continue drinking the meat stock and ginger tea. You can add some probiotic juices (sauerkraut, kim-chi, homemade kefir, and fermented vegetables) into every cup of meat stock and every bowl of soup. At this stage you can also begin adding raw organic egg yolks.

It was in this stage that I was able to start adding meats to my bone broth. You can add stews and casseroles made with meats and vegetables. You can also increase probiotic fermented foods and introduce fermented fish, starting from one piece a day and gradually increasing. You can also use 1 teaspoon of homemade ghee per day to begin with and gradually increase.

STAGE 3:

In this stage, you continue with all previous foods in Stage 1 and 2. You can now begin to add into soups 1-3 tsp of mashed ripe avocados. You can make pancakes from organic nut butters, eggs, and zucchini or squash. At this stage you can also eat scrambled eggs, fermented vegetables, and probiotics (bio-kult).

STAGE 4:

In Stage 4, you continue all of the foods introduced in the previous three stages, but gradually add in roasted or grilled meats. Begin adding a few drops of extra virgin olive oil to the meals and gradually increase the amount to 1-2 tablespoons per meal. Introduce a few spoonful's of freshly pressed carrot juice.

You can also add in gluten free nut breads, made from almond flour or other nut/seed flours.

STAGE 5:

Stage 5 continues with all previous foods and if you are tolerating everything in the previous four stages, you can add in cooked, puréed apples. This is the stage that you can now add raw vegetables starting from softer parts of lettuce and peeled cucumber. If the fresh pressed juices (carrot, celery, lettuce, mint) are well tolerated, start adding fruit (apple, pineapple, mango) if candida overgrowth is not a concern.

STAGE 6:

Continue all foods from the previous five stages. If you are tolerating all other foods well, you can begin to introduce some peeled, raw apple and other raw fruits and honey. After successfully introducing Stage 6 foods for several days with no digestive disruption, you may move to the full GAPS Diet.

Full GAPS Diet:

After completing the six stages, you can begin on the full GAPS Diet. For those who do not have severe digestive symptoms, food allergies, food intolerances, or irritable bowel syndrome (IBS), you can just skip the first six steps and move into the full GAPS diet. This is still a healing diet, but is for those who need less healing than people with severe intestinal disorders.

Sample Menu of Full GAPS diet:

When you wake up, begin with a glass of lemon water and/or fresh pressed vegetable juice with water added.

Breakfast:
- Eggs with runny yolk

181

- Sausage or other meats
- Vegetables, cooked or raw
- Avocado
- Cold pressed olive oil
- Soaked or sprouted nuts or seeds
- Nut flour Pancakes
- Nut flour muffins or bread
- A cup of warm meat stock to drink with your food
- Ginger or mint herbal teas
- Weak tea with lemon

Lunch & Dinner Options:

- Homemade vegetable soup or stew
- Meat, poultry, fish, or shellfish
- Vegetables, cooked or raw
- Avocado
- Olive oil with a squeeze of lemon as a dressing
- A cup of warm meat stock to drink with your food

These are the basic principles of the GAPS diet. I highly suggest reading The GAPS diet by Dr. Natasha Campbell McBride for a full list of allowed and not-allowed foods as well as recipes.

20

The Ketogenic Diet

The basic principles of the Ketogenic Diet are to increase the healthy fats and decrease the carbohydrates; which will eventually cause weight loss and increased health. This diet includes mostly vegetables, healthy fats and protein. The ketogenic diet was founded to help heal children with epilepsy when nothing else worked. However, the ketogenic diet was found to heal more than just epilepsy because you are feeding the body healthy fats, which reverses many diseases by restoring the electrical charge within the body.

"The ketogenic diet works on the principle that when no carbohydrate is stored in the muscles for energy, the body will power itself using its fat stores as its fuel source (a process called ketosis), which causes you to lose weight quickly, efficiently and safely." "To attain ketosis, you need to eat a diet that is very low in carbohydrate (may be as low as 20 grams per day). Your diet is based mostly on healthy fats, protein and green vegetables, which will make up most of the carbohydrates you consume but also giving you vital nutrients." (1).

This diet is complex at first because if you are really being strict about being on the ketogenic diet, you must weigh your food portions with a food scale and it needs to be precise measurements. After you have done this diet for a week, you begin to get used to measuring and can begin to easily tell how much of a specific food you can eat at one sitting without weighing each time. But in the beginning, you will need a food scale because you will be weighing each food item before you put it onto your plate and into your mouth.

The ketogenic diet varies on carbohydrate count depending upon whom you are reading. Some advocates of the ketogenic diet use total carb count and don't go above 20 grams of total carbohydrates per day. While other advocates of the ketogenic diet measure net carbs; which is carbohydrates minus fiber, and will vary their carb count from 20 – 30 net grams of carbs daily. I have personally found that I cannot go too low on carbohydrates as it makes me feel horrible, but I also have thyroid and adrenal issues. It really depends upon how the diet makes you feel when you are on it.

You are also allowed healthy fats on the ketogenic diet. There has long been a myth that eating fats will cause you to get fat, but nothing could be further from the truth. Eating healthy fats can actually help you to lose weight. Examples of healthy fats are coconut oil, olive oil, avocado oil, flax oil, walnut oil, grass fed butter, ghee, seeds and oils high in omega 3 fats. Coconut oil and Ghee are both high heat oils, which means that they are safe to cook with because you can heat it to high temperatures and the oil will stay stable. Olive Oil should only be used for cooking sparingly, but not over high heat. Olive Oil is great for drizzling over salads, vegetables and meats. You can also add more olives to your salads to increase your intake of healthy fats. Avocado oil is also great for salads or you can just eat more avocados daily to get the benefits of the high fat content. Walnut oil is great for salads or you can just add more walnuts to your daily routine. Make sure your walnuts are raw for the best health benefit.

Grass fed butter is wonderful and tastes so lovely. You can cook with real butter or use it as an accompaniment. My favorite butter is Kerry Gold salted butter which comes from the grass-fed cows of Ireland. I also sometimes enjoy butter from France, which is also churned from the cream of grass fed cows.

The Ketogenic diet not only helps with weight loss, but helps to stabilize insulin levels and diminish disease. An example of a day in the life of a ketogenic dieter:

Breakfast:

2 slices of turkey bacon or 2 eggs (scrambled in coconut oil).

17.5 grams of Sautéed spinach (sautéed in olive oil or coconut oil) or 15 grams of asparagus.

Lunch:

Hamburger Patty (60 grams)

½ Avocado (14 grams)

Dinner:

Turkey salad with crumbled blue cheese, tomato, ½ avocado and cucumber with an olive oil/balsamic vinegar dressing.

Or

Wild Salmon (60 grams) with Sautéed Asparagus Spears (15 grams)

Foods Allowed on the Ketogenic Diet:

- **Meat:** Any meat (such as beef, venison, pork, veal, lamb). Uncured meats need to check the carb count and processing first.

- **Poultry:** Any poultry (chicken, turkey, quail, duck etc.). Leave the skin on poultry to increase the fat content. Poultry must not be breaded or battered.

- **Fish and Shellfish:** They should be fresh with no added sugars. Again, it must not be breaded or battered.

- **Eggs:** Eggs become a staple when you are on a ketogenic diet. Eggs may be prepared any way.

- **Cheese:** Most types of cheese are suitable for a ketogenic diet, though they do contain some carbs, so make sure you include these in your daily carb count to ensure you stay below your daily carb limit.

- **Vegetables:** Vegetables will be the source of most of the carbs you eat, but you still need to choose the lowest carb vegetables with the best nutritional value. Green leafy vegetables are the best; such as, spinach, all kinds of lettuce, cabbage, watercress, brussels sprouts, and kale. You may also eat broccoli, cauliflower, celery, cucumber, asparagus, bean sprouts, radishes and more, but must strictly limit your intake of sugary vegetables like peppers, onions, tomatoes, and avoid starchy vegetables like potatoes or corn.

- **Nuts and Seeds:** eaten in moderation as a snack.

- **Oil, butter and cream:** butter, olive oil, ghee, and coconut oil can be used in cooking. You can also add walnut, flax, and avocado oils to salads.

- **Fresh herbs and dry spices:** can be used for flavor.
- **Mayonnaise and oil based salad dressings:** are usually OK, check the carb content on the bottle or make it homemade.

- **Artificial Sweeteners:** stevia and xylitol can be used in place of sugar.

I have utilized the ketogenic diet and other low carb diets throughout the past eight years. Although the low carb diets work well with weight loss at first, I feel that they do further harm to those who already suffer from hormonal issues, thyroid, and adrenal insufficiency. This diet did not work well for me and made me feel much worse in the long run. I had also consulted with a nutritionist who also informed me that she was not a big fan of low carb dieting because it can further alter women's hormonal function.

Although I am not a fan of low carb dieting, especially for those with hormonal, thyroid and adrenal issues, you can do a lesser version of the ketogenic diet utilizing 30-49 grams of net carbs per day and balancing your meals to balance blood sugar and balance hormonal function and still be able to lose weight, although you may not be in ketosis.

Again, you will have to be the judge and listen to your own body as to whether a diet is working well for you or not. Please make sure that you do not have any hormonal issues prior to beginning this diet as it may make the situation worse. It is advised to consult with a qualified physician or nutritionist before undertaking any dietary change.

21

Vegan vs. Vegetarian Diets

A vegetarian diet is free from animal products; such as, milk, dairy, and meat, but sometimes vegetarians will consume eggs and fish. If a vegetarian eats fish, they are labeled a pescetarian. Conversely; a vegan stays away from anything produced from an animal, which includes eggs, dairy, honey, and meat. The vegan diet consists of mainly vegetables and soy protein.

These dietary changes may be beneficial if healing from certain diseases, however they are not for everyone and the lack of protein from meat sources can drain some people of B vitamins, causing a vitamin and mineral deficiency. I had utilized this diet for a time and did not thrive while being vegan. Although eating vegetarian or vegan does work well for some.

Many vegans and vegetarians will replace the meat with meat substitutions found in supermarkets, but the problem with these meat substitutions is that they are made primarily of wheat gluten, soy, and other genetically modified ingredients. Not many of the meat substitutes are very healthy, so if you choose to enlist a vegetarian or vegan diet, please be mindful of the ingredients you are consuming and that they are free from genetically modified ingredients.

It is also important to pay close attention to your levels of nutrients as sometimes it is easy for those who are vegetarian or vegan to become deficient in certain nutrients due to the lack of meat and dairy products. The nutrients to consider in a vegetarian or vegan diet are:

- **Proteins:** Plant proteins alone can provide enough of the essential and non-essential amino acids, if caloric intake is high enough to meet energy needs.

- **Whole grains, legumes, vegetables, seeds and nuts:** all contain both essential and non-essential amino acids.
- **Soy protein:** has been shown to be equal to proteins of animal origin. Be mindful that soy is primarily genetically modified in the United States and some other countries, so if you are going to consume soy, make sure it is from a non-gmo source. The consumption of soy can also be estrogenic in some people as well, think man-boobs in men or estrogen dominance in women.
- **Iron:** vegetarians and vegans may experience a greater risk of iron deficiency than non-vegetarians. The richest sources of iron are found in red meat, liver, and egg yolks. However, dried beans, spinach, enriched products, brewer's yeast, and dried fruits are all good plant sources of iron.
- **Vitamin B-12:** This comes naturally only from animal sources. Vegans need a reliable source of vitamin B-12, which can be found in some fortified breakfast cereals, fortified soy beverages, some brands of nutritional (brewer's) yeast, and other foods (check the labels), as well as vitamin supplements.
- **Vitamin D:** Vegans should have a reliable source of vitamin D. Vegans who don't get much sunlight may need a D3 supplement.
- **Calcium:** Vegetable greens such as spinach, kale and broccoli, some legumes, and soybean products, are good sources of calcium from plants.
- **Zinc:** Zinc is needed for growth and development. Good plant sources include grains, nuts and legumes. Shellfish are an excellent source of zinc. Take care to select supplements containing no more than 15-18 mg zinc. Supplements containing 50 mg or more may lower HDL (good) cholesterol in some people.

22

Allergen Free Diets

Many people are allergic or intolerant to gluten and need to be on a gluten free diet. I remember when I finally decided to go gluten free back in 2007 and I printed out a list with all of the foods which contained gluten ingredients. I took the list to the grocery store and started reading all of the labels of all of the foods I was used to eating. I quickly found out that everything I was eating had gluten in it and everything in that grocery store had gluten in it as well. I was only in the store about 15 minutes before I got so upset and started crying, in the middle of the supermarket. You see, I felt so helpless, like I would never be able to eat anything again.

Of course, in the beginning, I went gluten free only to lose weight, which worked fabulous. However, it wasn't until a few years later when I developed severe leaky gut that I found I was allergic to gluten and had to cut it out for good. I have first-hand experience with making dietary changes and the frustration you feel with having to give up those foods you have become accustomed to, but I assure you that I will make that transition easy for you.

Below is a list of all of the unsafe ingredients which contain gluten, referenced from www.celiac.com. Get in the habit of taking the list to the store with you and reading the backs of labels. Eventually, you will become so good at reading labels that you will no longer need the list or need to read labels because you will inherently know whether or not a food is safe.

Unsafe Foods List (Gluten ingredients):

- Abyssinian Hard
- Wheat triticum
- durum
- Alcohol
- Atta Flour
- Barley Grass

191

- Barley
- Barley Malt
- Barley Stearyldimonium
- Beer (barley or wheat)
- Bleached Flour
- Bran
- Bread Flour
- Brewer's Yeast
- Brown Flour
- Bulgur
- Bulgur Wheat
- Cereal Binding
- Chilton
- Club Wheat
- Common Wheat
- Cookie Crumbs
- Cookie Dough
- Cookie Dough Pieces
- Couscous
- Crisped Rice
- Dinkle (Spelt)
- Disodium
- Wheatgermamido
- Peg-2
- Sulfosuccinate
- Durum wheat
- Edible Coatings, Films, and Starch
- Einkorn (Triticum monococcum)
- Emmer (Triticum dicoccon)
- Enriched Bleached Flour (any type)
- Farina and Farina Graham
- Farro
- Filler
- Flour (wheat)
- Fu (dried wheat gluten)
- Germ
- Groats (barley, wheat)
- Graham Flour
- Granary Flour
- Hard Wheat
- Heeng
- Hing
- Hordeum Vulgare Extract
- Hydroxypropyltrimonium
- Hydrolyzed Wheat Protein
- Hydroxypropyl
- Kamut (Pasta wheat)
- Kluski Pasta
- Maida (Indian wheat flour)
- Malt
- Malted Barley Flour
- Malted Milk
- Malt Extract
- Malt Syrup
- Malt Flavoring
- Malt Vinegar
- Macha Wheat
- Matza
- Matzah
- Matzo
- Matzo Semolina
- Meripro 711
- Mir
- Nishasta
- Oriental Wheat
- Orzo Pasta
- Pasta
- Pearl Barley
- Persian Wheat (Triticum carthlicum)
- Perungayam
- Poulard Wheat (Triticum turgidum)
- Polish Wheat (Triticum polonicum)

- Rice Malt (if barley or Koji are used)
- Roux
- Rusk
- Rye
- Seitan
- Semolina
- Soy Sauce (contains wheat)
- Sprouted Wheat
- Strong Flour
- Suet in Packets
- Shot Wheat)
- Small Spelt
- Spirits (specific types)
- Spelt (Triticum spelta)
- Triticum
- Triticale X
- Tabbouleh
- Tabouli
- Teriyaki Sauce
- Timopheevi Wheat
- triticosecale
- Triticum Vulgare
- Udon (wheat noodles)
- Unbleached Flour
- Vavilovi Wheat
- Vital Wheat Gluten
- Wheat, Abyssinian Hard triticum durum
- Wheat Amino Acids
- Wheat Bran Extract
- Wheat, Bulgur
- Wheat Durum
- Wheat Germ Extract
- Wheat Germ Glycerides
- Wheat Germ Oil
- Wheat Germamidopropyl
- Wheat Grass (can contain seeds)
- Wheat Nuts
- Wheat Protein
- Wheat Triticum
- Wheat Triticum
- Wheat Bran Extract
- Whole-Meal Flour
- Wild Einkorn
- Wild Emmer

Due to the increasing amount of people who are allergic and intolerant to gluten, grocery stores have been catching on and now many of the grocery chains will carry gluten free foods. However, even when a food says that they are gluten free, it still may not be safe to consume because even the gluten free foods may contain genetically modified ingredients and other allergens.

Many people that are allergic or intolerant to gluten may also have multiple food sensitivities to other ingredients. So, even with the gluten free foods, you still need to read the labels to make sure they are free from other allergens and free from genetically modified ingredients. I had to stop eating all processed foods, even gluten free varieties, because they also contained soy, dairy, or corn, which I was also intolerant too. Below is a list of genetically modified ingredients, referenced from www.responsibletechnology.org, that are hidden in foods so you can be aware. Again, take this list to the super market and begin checking the labels, after a while, you will not need to check labels because it will become second nature to you.

Genetically Modified Ingredients (GMOs):

- Aspartame
- Amino Sweet ®
- Nutra Sweet ®
- Equal Spoonful ®
- Canderel ®
- BeneVia ®
- E951
- Baking powder
- canola oil
- Caramel color
- Cellulose
- Citric acid
- Cobalamin (vitamin B12)
- Colorose
- Condensed milk
- Confectioners' sugar
- Corn flour
- Corn masa
- Corn meal
- Corn oil
- Corn sugar
- Corn syrup
- Cornstarch
- Cottonseed oil
- Cysteine
- Cyclodextrin
- Dextrin
- Dextrose
- Diacetyl
- diglyceride
- Erythritol
- Equal
- Food starch
- Fructose (any form)
- Glucose
- Glutamate
- Glutamic acid
- Glycerides
- Glycerin
- Glycerol
- Glycerol monooleate
- Glycine
- Hemicellulose
- High fructose corn syrup (HFCS)
- Hydrogenated starch
- Hydrolyzed vegetable protein
- Inositol
- Inverse syrup
- Inversol
- Invert sugar
- Isoflavones
- Lactic acid
- lecithin
- Leucine
- Lysine
- Malitol
- Malt

- Malt syrup
- Malt extract
- Maltodextrin
- Maltose
- Mannitol
- Methylcellulose
- Milk powder
- Milo starch
- Modified food starch
- Modified starch
- Mono and diglycerides
- Monosodium glutamate (MSG)
- NutraSweet
- Oleic acid
- Phenylalanine
- Phytic acid
- Protein isolate
- Rapeseed oil
- Shoyu
- Sorbitol
- Soy flour
- Soy isolates
- Soy lecithin
- Soy milk
- Soy oil
- Soy protein
- Soy protein isolate
- Soy sauce
- Starch
- Stearic acid
- Sugar (unless cane sugar)
- Tamari
- tempeh
- Teriyaki marinades
- Textured vegetable protein
- Tofu
- threonine
- tocopherols (vitamin E)
- Trehalose
- Triglyceride
- Vegetable fat
- Vegetable oil
- Vitamin B12
- Vitamin C (ascorbic acid, derived from corn in the US).
- Vitamin E
- Whey
- Whey powder
- Xanthan gum

Many foods are now donning the gluten free, non-GMO, and vegan labels to make it easier for you to decipher through the mess that has become supermarket shopping and eating of the twenty-first century. No longer can we just go to the supermarket and buy the food off the shelves. Shopping now takes much longer because we are forced to read the labels, since our food is harming our children and families. Who would have ever thought that shopping for food, a basic source of life, would become so complex?

The easiest way to eat gluten free and allergen free is just to go back to eating fresh, whole foods in their base forms. Fresh organic vegetables, fresh organic meats, fresh organic fruits and make your own foods from scratch. I know that many people are pressed for time, as I am too, which is why my crock pot is my best friend. I use my crock pot all the time, throw in all of the ingredients in the morning and turn it on. It takes no more than 15 minutes to prepare the meal and let the crock pot do the rest.

With the knowledge from this book and a little practice, you will be able to master supermarket food shopping like a pro and not have to worry about feeding your family toxic ingredients because you are now armed with the knowledge of how to avoid harmful ingredients.

23

Low FODMAP Diet

After trying many dietary changes, I also had to enlist a low fodmap dietary change to deal with the food intolerances I was experiencing. What are FODMAPS you ask? FODMAP stands for Fermentable Oligosaccharides, Disaccharides, Monosaccharides, And Polyols. According to the Journal of Gastroenterology; FODMAPs are short-chain carbohydrates which are not completely absorbed in the gastrointestinal tract, which can then be easily fermented by the bacteria in the gut. (2). When these foods are ingested, they will turn into fermentable sugars which increase fluid movement into the large bowel. This is a major cause of irritable bowel syndrome (IBS) with diarrhea, gas, pain and bloating. (1).

Many people who suffer from food allergies, food intolerances, irritable bowel syndrome (IBS), irritable bowel disease (IBD), Crohn's disease, ulcerative colitis, intestinal permeability (leaky gut), and small intestinal bacterial overgrowth (SIBO) may benefit from staying away from high FODMAP foods and enlisting a diet of low residue FODMAPs. Below are two lists of the foods to avoid and foods you can eat when on a FODMAP diet (referenced from www.ibsgroup.org).

Foods to Avoid on FODMAP:

- **Fructose:** pear, canned fruit, watermelon, apple, mango, dried fruit, fruit juice, fructose, high fructose corn syrup, honey.
- **Lactose:** milks and cheeses; cow, goat, sheep, ice cream, yogurt, custard, cottage cheese, cream cheese, soft unripened cheeses, ricotta, mascarpone.

- **Fructans:** Vegetables; cabbage, shallots, onions, leeks, garlic, okra, fennel, brussels sprouts, asparagus, artichokes, broccoli, beets. Cereals; wheat, rye, cookies, crackers, couscous, pasta. Miscellaneous; dandelion, chicory, inulin, pistachio.
- **Galactans:** Legumes; chickpeas, lentils, kidney beans, soy beans, baked beans.
- **Polyols:** Fruits; watermelon, cherry, peach, pear, plum, prune, apple, apricot, avocado, blackberry, lychee, nashi, nectarine, longon. Vegetables; mushrooms, green bell peppers, corn, cauliflower. Sweetener; xylitol, sorbitol, mannitol, isomalt, maltitol.

Foods Suitable on Low FODMAP:

- **Fruits:** banana, blueberry, strawberry, tangelo, star anise, rock melon, rhubarb, raspberry, passion fruit, mandarin orange, cantaloupe, durian, grapes, honeydew, grapefruit, cranberry, kiwi, lemons, limes.
- **Vegetables:** sweet potato, yam, zucchini, squash, taro, tomato, alfalfa, bamboo shoots, bok choy, celery, carrots, choy sum, ginger, eggplant, choko, endive, green beans, lettuce, red bell pepper, silver beet, pumpkin, potato, parsnip, olives, spinach.
- **Herbs:** rosemary, thyme, parsley, oregano, basil, chili, coriander, ginger, lemongrass, mint, marjoram.
- **Grains:** gluten free bread, 100% spelt bread, gluten free cereals, gluten free oats, rice, polenta, arrowroot, millet, psyllium, quinoa, tapioca, sorghum.
- **Dairy:** lactose free milk, oat milk, rice milk, almond milk, brie, camembert, hard cheeses, non-dairy or lactose free yogurt, sorbet, non-dairy ice cream.
- **Other:** organic tofu, stevia, olive oil.

24

Extend Your Faith

One of the major reasons that I overcame this very long trial of chronic illness, which led me to the path of wellness, is only partially attributed to changing my diet and detoxification. A path to wellness is also attributed to my belief, extreme faith, and trust in God. Going through the trials of life is usually when people are closest to God and turn to God for answers. During my crisis, I prayed daily, mostly hourly, and mostly through tears, that God would lead me to a treatment that would heal me of any disease lurking within my body. I had to completely give my life over to God and trust in him completely that he would heal me and lead me in the right direction.

While I was going through cancer, I figured that if it was my time to die than I was fine with that because I am a Christian and I knew that I would go to Heaven. I also believed that it didn't matter where I was; whether it is in a hospital or at home, that if God wanted to heal me of cancer or other diseases than he would do so, as long as I took responsibility for my own health and was proactive in my healing. So, I gave my life to God and am comfortable with my decision to forego doctors, hospitals, mutilating surgery, needles, and toxic drugs. Although, when I did begin to go back to doctors for testing, I found that the stress of the procedures and ignorance of doctors had made my health conditions much worse. I am not telling everyone to forego doctors as there may be some good doctors out there, I just haven't found any.

I made it a point to heal the way God intended, with the natural, organic plants, and seeds that he had created for us to utilize for health. Everything on this earth was created by God and he created everything with healing in mind. It just takes time to find the right cure for each disease. I now realize that most every disease and illness is reversible using only alternative methods, which are actually the original methods in which God created. I have come to this conclusion through my own trial of cancer and other major health issues, extensive research, experimentation, and healing.

It was also imperative for me to be close to the Lord, which is why I found myself praying constantly throughout the day just to stay strong. There were so many times throughout the day that I would break into tears and feel a deep despair. I learned later that tears are just another way of your body doing the necessary house cleaning and detoxification of your system, so cry all you want as it is good for you to get it out.

As my faith grew, I began thanking God in advance for my healing and turning my situation around. I expected God to be good to me and I prayed as if the Lord had already blessed me. The more I prayed and thanked God for his blessings, the more I received blessings. I ended up moving to a new location which I felt would be healthier for me. I kept praying for God to bring me friends in my new location and within a couple of months of moving, I met a neighbor who invited me to her church to view the movie; "War Room."

My faith in God has helped me through these trials of illness and I know that God will help you as well, just ask him, he will not forsake you. Find a good church and a church support group to help you through your trial as well, it really helps to increase your faith and bring you closer to God.

Through this extremely long trial of illness and poverty, I had faced long-term unemployment multiple times, cancer twice, deathbed once, chronic inflammation, chronic disease, extreme poverty, welfare/food stamps, and betrayal of so-called friends and family, personal hate-filled verbal attacks, hate mail, and family turmoil. Through it all, God still gave me enough healthy food to eat and a roof over my head while I was healing my body. I realized that God kept pressing on my heart, telling me to write my first book on healing cancer and this book about detoxification, to help others who are sick and also in despair and to get the truth out about how to heal the body naturally, God's way.

It seemed as if the longer I kept putting off finishing this book, the more horrible things kept happening to me, until I followed what God wanted me to do. Satan kept attacking me and the more I procrastinated, the more I felt a knot deep in the pit of my stomach and unrest because I knew that God had opened the door for me to write this book and I was supposed to finish it. During this eight plus year trial in my life, I really felt a kinship with the book of Job and his trials because my own trials were taking on a tragically similar course, although they had lasted much longer.

It is so easy to become lazy and complacent, especially when you are chronically ill, not feeling well, and trying to heal, but I had to put my best foot forward to finish this book for the Lord and hopefully to help someone in the process. Exodus 23:25 states, "Worship the Lord your God, and his blessing will be on your food and water. I will take away sickness from among you." (NLT).

Healing Scriptures:

It helps to remain positive through your illness and believe that you will be healed. Even though you may be very weary and feeling hopeless, it is imperative that you boost your spirit and faith by reading the bible, praying daily, or even hourly if needed, and focus upon giving your troubles to the Lord, and having faith that he will heal you.

The following Healing Scriptures are here to help you to increase your faith. When you are chronically ill and feel despair, you can open to this chapter and begin reading these healing scriptures and repeat them to yourself daily to increase your faith in the Lord for your complete healing.

Psalm 30:2 O Lord my God, I cried out to you for help, and you restored my health.
James 5:15 And their prayer offered in faith will heal the sick, and the Lord will make them well. And anyone who has committed sins will be forgiven.
Matthew 4:23 Jesus traveled throughout Galilee teaching in the synagogues, preaching everywhere the Good News about the Kingdom. And he healed people who had every kind of sickness and disease.

Matthew 8:17 This fulfilled the word of the Lord through Isaiah, who said, "He took our sicknesses and removed our diseases."

Luke 4:18 The Spirit of the Lord is upon me, for he has appointed me to preach Good News to the poor. He has sent me to proclaim that captives will be released, that the blind will see, that the downtrodden will be freed from their oppressors.

Psalm 103:2-3 Praise the Lord, I tell myself, and never forget the good things he does for me. He forgives all my sins and heals all my diseases.

Romans 8:26 And the Holy Spirit helps us in our distress. For we don't even know what we should pray for, nor how we should pray. But the Holy Spirit prays for us with groaning that cannot be expressed in words.

Luke 7:21 At that very time, he cured many people of their various diseases, and he cast out evil spirits and restored sight to the blind.

Isaiah 35:5-6 And when he comes, he will open the eyes of the blind and unstop the ears of the deaf. The lame will leap like a deer, and those who cannot speak will shout and sing! Springs will gush forth in the wilderness, and streams will water the desert.

Matthew 21:14 The blind and the lame came to him, and he healed them there in the Temple.

Exodus 15:26 If you will listen carefully to the voice of the Lord your God and do what is right in his sight, obeying his commands and laws, then I will not make you suffer the diseases I sent on the Egyptians; for I am the Lord who heals you.

Psalm 91:14-16 The Lord says, "I will rescue those who love me. I will protect those who trust in my name. When they call on me, I will answer; I will be with them in trouble. I will rescue them and honor them. I will satisfy them with a long life and give them my salvation."

Psalm 50:15 Trust me in your times of trouble, and I will rescue you, and you will give me glory.

Luke 1:37 For nothing is impossible with God.

Matthew 9:35 Jesus traveled through all the cities and villages of that area, teaching in the synagogues and announcing the Good News about the Kingdom. And wherever he went, he healed people of every sort of disease and illness.

Acts 3:6 But Peter said, "I don't have any money for you. But I'll give you what I have. In the name of Jesus Christ of Nazareth, get up and walk!"

Isaiah 32:3-4 Then everyone who can see will be looking for God, and those who can hear will listen to his voice. Even the hotheads among them will be full of sense and understanding. Those who stammer in uncertainty will speak out plainly.

Matthew 20:34 Jesus felt sorry for them and touched their eyes. Instantly they could see! Then they followed him.

Psalm 91:9-10 If you make the Lord your refuge, if you make the Most High your shelter, no evil will conquer you; no plague will come near your dwelling.

Isaiah 53:4-5 Yet it was our weaknesses he carried; it was our sorrows that weighed him down. And we thought his troubles were a punishment from God for his own sins! But he was wounded and crushed for our sins. He was beaten that we might have peace. He was whipped, and we were healed!

Mark 8:25 Then Jesus placed his hands over the man's eyes again. As the man stared intently, his sight was completely restored, and he could see everything clearly.

Psalm 34:17-19 The Lord hears his people when they call to him for help. He rescues them from all their troubles. The Lord is close to the brokenhearted; he rescues those who are crushed in spirit. The righteous face many troubles, but the Lord rescues them from each and every one.

Galatians 3:14 Through the work of Christ Jesus, God has blessed the Gentiles with the same blessing he promised to Abraham, and we Christians receive the promised Holy Spirit through faith.

Isaiah 58:8 If you do these things, your salvation will come like the dawn. Yes, your healing will come quickly. Your godliness will lead you forward, and the glory of the Lord will protect you from behind.

Isaiah 40:31 But those who wait on the Lord will find new strength. They will fly high on wings like eagles. They will run and not grow weary. They will walk and not faint.

Acts 14:9-10 He was listening as Paul preached, and Paul noticed him and realized he had faith to be healed. So Paul called to him in a loud voice, "Stand up!" And the man jumped to his feet and started walking.

Matthew 8:2-3 Suddenly, a man with leprosy approached Jesus. He knelt before him, worshiping, "Lord," the man said, "if you want to, you can make me well again." Jesus touched him. "I want to," he said. "Be healed!" And instantly the leprosy disappeared.

Proverbs 14:30 A relaxed attitude lengthens life; jealousy rots it away.

Isaiah 57:19 Then words of praise will be on their lips. May they have peace; both near and far, for I will heal them all, says the Lord.

Romans 8:2 For the power of the life-giving Spirit has freed you through Christ Jesus for the power of sin that leads to death.

Luke 4:40 As the sun went down that evening, people throughout the village brought sick family members to Jesus. No matter what their diseases were, the touch of his hand healed everyone.

Proverbs 17:22 A cheerful heart is good medicine, but a broken spirit saps a person's strength.

Psalm 147:3 He heals the brokenhearted, binding up their wounds.

Proverbs 16:24 Kind words are like honey-sweet to the soul and healthy for the body.

I Peter 2:24 He personally carried away our sins in his own body on the cross so we can be dead to sin and live for what is right. You have been healed by his wounds!

3 John 2 Dear friend, I am praying that all is well with you and that your body is as healthy as I know your soul is.

Acts 10:38 And no doubt you know that God anointed Jesus of Nazareth with the Holy Spirit and with power. Then Jesus went around doing good and healing all who were oppressed by the Devil, for God was with him.

Proverbs 11:17 Your own soul is nourished when you are kind, but you destroy yourself when you are cruel.

Proverbs 3:7-8 Don't be impressed with your own wisdom. Instead, fear the Lord and turn your back on evil. Then you will gain renewed health and vitality.

Psalm 42:11 Why am I discouraged? Why so sad? I will put my hope in God! I will praise him again-my Savior and my God!

Exodus 23:25 "You must serve only the Lord your God. If you do, I will bless you with food and water, and I will keep you healthy.

Malachi 4:2 "But for you who fear my name, the Sun of Righteousness will rise with healing in his wings. And you will go free, leaping with joy like calves let out to pasture.

II Chronicles 30:20 And the Lord listened to Hezekiah's prayer and healed the people.

Matthew 15:30-31 A vast crowd brought him the lame, blind, crippled, mute, and many others with physical difficulties, and they laid them before Jesus. And he healed them all.

Matthew 8:16 That evening many demon-possessed people were brought to Jesus. All the spirits fled when he commanded them to leave; and he healed all the sick.

Luke 9: 2, 6 Then he sent them out to tell everyone about the coming of the Kingdom of God and to heal the sick. So they began their circuit of the villages, preaching the good News and healing the sick.

Isaiah 33:24 The people of Israel will no longer say, "We are sick and helpless," for the Lord will forgive their sins.

Deuteronomy 7:15 And the Lord will protect you from all sickness. He will not let you suffer from the terrible diseases you knew in Egypt, but he will bring them all on your enemies!

Psalm 107:20 He spoke, and they were healed-snatched from the door of death.

Proverbs 4:20-22 Pay attention, my child, to what I say. Listen carefully. Don't lose sight of my words. Let them penetrate deep within your heart, for they bring life and radiant health to anyone who discovers their meaning.

Matthew 12:22 Then a demon-possessed man, who was both blind and unable to talk, was brought to Jesus. He healed the man so that he could both speak and see.

Acts 5:16 Crowds came in from the villages around Jerusalem, bringing their sick and those possessed by evil spirits, and they were all healed.

Isaiah 29:18 In that day deaf people will hear words read from a book, and blind people will see through the gloom and darkness.

Matthew 9:29-30 Then he touched their eyes and said, "Because of your faith, it will happen." And suddenly they could see! Jesus sternly warned them, "Don't tell anyone about this."

Matthew 9:20-22 a woman who had a hemorrhage for twelve years came up behind him. She touched the fringe of his robe, for she thought, "If I can just touch his robe, I will be healed." Jesus turned around and said to her, "Daughter be encouraged! Your faith has made you well." And the woman was healed at that moment.

Mark 10:52 And Jesus said to him, "Go your way. Your faith has healed you." And instantly the blind man could see! Then he followed Jesus down the road.

25

Conclusion

I sincerely hope that this book has touched your soul to begin to help yourself and learn to heal your body the way God intended. Through my journey of chronic illness, discovery of the root cause of disease, and complete healing, I pray that you have found the information in this book to be invaluable to you and your family's health in how to heal through God's Pharmacy. Unfortunately, with much of the world having a socialist, universal healthcare system, we are not getting the kind of healthcare that we deserve and you will never heal if you are taking pills from the pharmaceutical companies that do nothing but mask your symptoms, never dealing with the root cause of your health problem.

My advice to you is to clean up your diet, detoxify your body regularly, and learn to listen to the symptoms in your body so you can learn to heal yourself. It is imperative to take your health into your own hands as nobody will do it for you. Once you begin to detoxify your body from the overabundance of toxins, it will become easier to listen to your body and to know what is going on. There comes an inner wisdom, an internal knowledge, only found through proper detoxification and eating clean. By following the principles in this book, you will tap into a greater health and sensitivity that you could ever imagine.

Take great care of your body to help yourself heal naturally and know that "You can achieve optimum health through God's pharmacy."

References

Chapter 1: Feeling Like "Job"
1. St. John, T. (2013). Defeat Cancer Now. California.
Alternative Health Solutions.

Chapter 2: Why Are We Sick?
1. Basic Information about Fluoride in Drinking Water. (2012.
May 21). Retrieved from United States Environmental
Protection Agency Website:
http://water.epa.gov/drink/contaminants/basicinformation/fluo
ride.cfm
2. Group, E. The Dangers of Fluoride. (2009. March 26).
Retrieved from Global Healing Center Website.
http://www.globalhealingcenter.com/natural-health/how-safe-
is-fluoride
3. Miller, D. Fluoride Follies (n.d.) Retrieved from Tetrahedron
Publishing Group Website.
http://www.tetrahedron.org/articles/health_risks/fluoride_follie
s.html
4. Smith, J. (n.d.) What is a GMO. Retrieved from The
Institute for Responsible Technology Website.
www.responsibletechnology.org
5. President's Cancer Panel Warns Public of Chemical Dangers.
(n.d.) Retrieved from Environmental Working Group Website.
http://www.ewg.org/chemindex/term/510
6. National Drinking Water Database. (2009 December).
Retrieved from Environmental Working Group Website.
http://www.ewg.org/tap-water/executive-summary
7. Persistent Bioaccumulative and Toxic (PBT) Chemical
Program. (n.d.). Retrieved from Environmental Protection
Agency Website. http://www.epa.gov/pbt/pubs/ddt.htm
8. Smith, J. State of the Science on the Health Risks of GM
Foods (2010 February 15). Retrieved from Institute for
Responsible Technology Website.
http://www.responsibletechnology.org/docs/145.pdf
9. The Disgusting Symptoms of Agent Orange (Dioxin)
Poisoning. (2011. May 9). Retrieved from Vets Helping Vets
Website. http://www.myveteran.org/2011/05/agent-orange-
symptoms.html
10. National Cancer Act of 1971. (n.d.). Retrieved from The
National Cancer Institute Website.

http://dtp.nci.nih.gov/timeline/noflash/milestones/M4_Nixon.ht
m
11. Campbell, C. & Campbell T. (2006). The China Study.
Texas: Benbella Books.
12. Whitmont, Ron. 2015. "Chronic Illness and the Human
Microbiome." *American Journal of Homeopathic Medicine* 108,
no. 3: 115-123. *Alt HealthWatch*, EBSCO*host* (accessed
January 14, 2016).
13. St. John, T. (2013). Defeat Cancer Now. California.
Alternative Health Solutions.

Chapter 3: Why Detoxification?

1. St. John, T. (2013). Defeat Cancer Now. California.
Alternative Health Solutions.

Chapter 4: Testing Methods

1. Information & HCG Urine Test. (n.d.). Retrieved from
Navarro Medical Clinic Website. www.navarromedicalclinic.com
2. Cantwell, A. (1983). AIDS; The Mystery & The Solution.
California: Aries Rising Press.
3. Harter Pierce, T. (2000). Outsmart Your Cancer;
Alternative Non-Toxic Treatments That Work. Nevada:
Thoughtworks Publishing.
4. Fischer, W. (2000). How to Fight Cancer and Win.
Maryland: Agora Health Books.
5. St. John, T. (2013). Defeat Cancer Now. California.
Alternative Health Solutions.
6. Sarandakou, Angeliki, Efthimia Protonotariou, and
Demetrios Rizos. 2007. "Tumor Markers In Biological Fluids
Associated With Pregnancy". *Critical Reviews in Clinical
Laboratory Sciences.* 44 (2): 151-178.
7. Liao, Xing-Hua, Yue Wang, Nan Wang, Ting-Bao Yan, Wen-
Jing Xing, Li Zheng, Dong-Wei Zhao, et al. 2014. "Human
chorionic gonadotropin decreases human breast cancer cell
proliferation and promotes differentiation". *IUBMB Life.* 66 (5):
352-360.
8. Lab Tests Plus Website. www.labtestsplus.com
9. UniKey Health Website. www.unikeyhealth.com
10. 23 and Me Genetic Testing Website. www.23andme.com
11. Genetic Genie Website. http://geneticgenie.org

Chapter 5: Barriers to Detoxification

1. How to Heal Leaky Gut, Alternative Health Solutions Website. Written on December 8, 2014. http://tamarastjohn.com/how-to-heal-leaky-gut/ Accessed on January 18, 2016.
2. Licorice (*Glycyrrhiza glabra* L.) and DGL (deglycyrrhizinated licorice). National Center for Complimentary and Integrative Health Web site. Accessed at https://nccih.nih.gov/health/licoriceroot on January 26, 2016.
3. Herb Wisdom website. Licorice Root http://www.herbwisdom.com/herb-licorice-root.html Accessed January 30, 2016.
4. Herb Wisdom Website Slippery Elm http://www.herbwisdom.com/herb-slippery-elm.html Accessed on January 30, 2016.
5. Briden, Lara, ND. Lara Briden's Healthy Hormone Blog. Written January 12, 2016. http://www.larabriden.com/the-curious-link-between-estrogen-and-histamine-intolerance Accessed January 12, 2016.
6. Updated on February 2, 2015 by: Emily Wax, RD, The Brooklyn Hospital Center, Brooklyn, NY. Also reviewed by David Zieve, MD, MHA, Isla Ogilvie, PhD, and the A.D.A.M. Editorial team. https://www.nlm.nih.gov/medlineplus/ency/article/002402.htm Accessed on January 12, 2016.

Chapter 6: The Colon Cleanse

1. Colbert, D. (2000). Toxic Relief. Florida: Siloam Press.
2. Herbal Parasite Killing Cleanse. (n.d.). Retrieved from Dr. Clark's Legacy Website. http://www.drhuldaclark.org/herbal-parasite-killing-cleanse
3. Liver Cleanse. (n.d.). Retrieved from Dr. Clark's Legacy Website. http://www.drhuldaclark.org/liver-cleanse
4. Coffee Enemas Reverses Cancer; By Waste Removal and Detoxifying. (n.d.). Treating Cancer Alternatively Website, Retrieved from http://www.treating-cancer-alternatively.com/Coffee-enemas.html
5. What is Candida. (n.d.). Retrieved from The Candida Diet Website. http://www.thecandidadiet.com
6. Wilson, L. Coffee Enemas: History & Benefits. (2012. April 21). Retrieved from Healing AIA Holistic Website. http://www.healingaia.com/blog-resources/nutritional-balancing/five-elements-of-nutritional-balancing/detox-protocols/coffee-enemas

7. Cairo, M. & Bishop, M. (2004). Tumour lysis syndrome: new therapeutic strategies and classification. British Journal of Haematology, 127: 3–11. doi: 10.1111/j.1365-2141.2004. 05094.x, Retrieved from Wiley Online Library Website http://onlinelibrary.wiley.com/doi/10.1111/j.1365-2141.2004.05094.x/full

8. Harter Pierce, T. (2000). Outsmart Your Cancer; Alternative Non-Toxic Treatments That Work. Nevada: Thoughtworks Publishing.

9. St. John, T. (2013). Defeat Cancer Now; A Nutritional Approach to Wellness for Cancer and Other Diseases. California: Alternative Health Solutions.

10. The Benefits of Triphala for Hair, Skin, and Cleansing. Superfood Profiles. http://superfoodprofiles.com/triphala-benefits-health Accessed January 19, 2016.

11. Triphala. MD Health. Com http://www.md-health.com/Triphala.html Accessed January 19, 2016.

Chapter 7: The Candida Cleanse

1. Colbert, D. (2000). Toxic Relief. Florida: Siloam Press.

2. Herbal Parasite Killing Cleanse. (n.d.). Retrieved from Dr. Clark's Legacy Website http://www.drhuldaclark.org/herbal-parasite-killing-cleanse

3. Liver Cleanse. (n.d.). Retrieved from Dr. Clark's Legacy Website. http://www.drhuldaclark.org/liver-cleanse

4. Coffee Enemas Reverses Cancer; By Waste Removal and Detoxifying. (n.d.). Treating Cancer Alternatively Website, Retrieved from http://www.treating-cancer-alternatively.com/Coffee-enemas.html

5. What is Candida. (n.d.). Retrieved from The Candida Diet Website. http://www.thecandidadiet.com

6. Wilson, L. Coffee Enemas: History & Benefits. (2012. April 21). Retrieved from Healing AIA Holistic Website. http://www.healingaia.com/blog-resources/nutritional-balancing/five-elements-of-nutritional-balancing/detox-protocols/coffee-enemas

7. Cairo, M. & Bishop, M. (2004). Tumour lysis syndrome: new therapeutic strategies and classification. British Journal of Haematology, 127: 3–11. doi: 10.1111/j.1365-2141.2004. 05094.x, Retrieved from Wiley Online Library Website. http://onlinelibrary.wiley.com/doi/10.1111/j.1365-2141.2004.05094.x/full

8. Harter Pierce, T. (2000). Outsmart Your Cancer; Alternative Non-Toxic Treatments That Work. Nevada: Thoughtworks Publishing.

9. Boroch, Ann. (2009). The Candida Cure; Yeast, Fungus, and your Health. Los Angeles, California: Quintessential Healing Publishing, Inc.
10. St. John, T. (2013). Defeat Cancer Now; A Nutritional Approach to Wellness for Cancer and Other Diseases. California: Alternative Health Solutions.
11.Herb Wisdom Website. Oregano. http://www.herbwisdom.com/herb-oregano.html Accessed on January 30, 2016.
12. Applied Health Website. http://appliedhealth.com/benefits-of-grapefruit-seed-extract Accessed on January 30, 2016.
13. Herbs 2000 Website. http://www.herbs2000.com/herbs/herbs_pau_darco.htm Accessed on January 30, 2016.
14. Wong, Cathy. ND. Altmedicine website last updated January 14, 2016. http://altmedicine.about.com/od/coconutoil/a/Caprylic-Acid.htm   Accessed on January 30, 2016.
15. Crook, William G. MD. The Yeast Connection. Vintage Books, New York. 1986.
16. Herb Wisdom website. http://www.herbwisdom.com/herb-olive-leaf.html   Accessed on January 30, 2016.
17. The Candida Diet Website. http://www.thecandidadiet.com/oregongrapes.htm   Accessed on January 30, 2016.
18. Mountain Rose Herbs website. https://www.mountainroseherbs.com/products/oregon-grape-root-extract/profile   Accessed on January 29, 2016.
19. Home Remedy Central Website. Oregon Grape Root Extract. http://www.homeremedycentral.com/en/herbal-remedies/extracts/oregon-grape-root-extract.html   Accessed on January 29, 2016.
20. Herb Wisdom.Com website. Herbal Benefits. http://www.herbwisdom.com/herb-goldenseal.html   Accessed on January 29, 2016.
 21. Weiss, Janice. http://www.candidapage.com/aldehyde.shtml Retrieved on January 6, 2016.

Chapter 8: Those Nasty Parasites

1. ZACCONE P, FEHERVARI Z, PHILLIPS JM, DUNNE DW, COOKE A. Parasitic worms and inflammatory diseases. *Parasite Immunology*. 2006;28(10):515-523. doi:10.1111/j.1365-3024.2006.00879.x.

2. Alex A. Volinsky a*, Nikolai V. Gubarev b, Galina M. Orlovskaya c, Elena V. Marchenko. Human anaerobic intestinal "rope" parasites. Cornell University Library.
3. Steven D. Ehrlich, NMD. http://umm.edu/health/medical/altmed/condition/roundworms. University of Maryland Medical Center. Reviewed on December 9, 2014. Accessed on December 21, 2015.
4. Joseph Sylvester, Neem, The Village Pharmacy. Accessed on December 29, 2015. http://www.netowne.com/alt-healing/ayurveda
5. Global Healing Center, http://superfoodprofiles.com/pumpkin-seeds-parasites-intestinal-worms. Accessed January 12, 2016.
6. Tapeworms in Humans. http://www.webmd.com/digestive-disorders/tapeworms-in-humans. Accessed January 16, 2016.
7. Murat Hökelek, MD, PhD. "Nematode Infections." Medscape. http://emedicine.medscape.com/article/224011-overview   Accessed January 17, 2016.
8. Subhash Chandra Parija, MBBS, MD, PhD, FRCPath, DSc. "Trematode Infection." Medscape. http://emedicine.medscape.com/article/230112-overview Accessed January 17, 2016.
9. Pinnacle Health and Wellness. Article published September 28, 2012. http://www.wellness24.org/fluke-parasites-the-intestinal-human-parasite-a-61.html Accessed January 17, 2016.
10. Dr. Clark Information Center. http://www.drclark.net/the-essentials/advanced/parasites-advanced/we-all-have-parasites Accessed January 17, 2016.
11. The University of Texas Medical Branch at Galveston. 1996. http://www.ncbi.nlm.nih.gov/books/NBK8037 Accessed January 17, 2016.
12. WebMD http://www.webmd.com/vitamins-supplements/ingredientmono-577-NEEM.aspx?activeIngredientId=577&activeIngredientName=NEEM   Accessed January 17, 2016.
13. Wolf Creek Ranch Animal Sanctuary. http://wolfcreekranch1.tripod.com/diatomaceous_earth.html Accessed January 17, 2016.
14. Human Parasite Symptoms. Diatomaceous Earth, Humans, and Parasites. Written on April 27, 2010. http://www.humanparasitesymptoms.com/human-tapeworm/diatomaceous-earth-humans-parasites   Accessed on January 17, 2016.

15. Herbal Extract Plus Website.
http://www.herbalextractsplus.com/pumpkin-seed.html
Accessed on January 18, 2016.
16. Ehrlich, Steven D., NMD. University of Maryland Medical
Center Website. Reviewed April 8, 2014.
http://umm.edu/health/medical/altmed/condition/intestinal-
parasites   Accessed on January 18, 2016.
17. Centers for Disease Control and Prevention. Giardia.
http://www.cdc.gov/parasites/giardia/index.html Accessed on
January 26, 2016.
18. Centers for Disease Control and Prevention.
http://www.cdc.gov/parasites/resources/pdf/npi_factsheet.pdf
Accessed on January 26, 2016.
19. Natural Vitality Center Website.
http://www.nvcentre.com/nvc2003/uni_symptoms_paras.php
Accessed on January 30, 2016.
20. Ferger, Jessica. CBS Website. CDC Warns of Common
Parasite Plaguing Millions in US. Published May 8, 2014.
http://www.cbsnews.com/news/parasites-causing-infections-
in-the-us-cdc-says   Accessed on January 30, 2016.
21. Herb Wisdom Website. Cloves.
http://www.herbwisdom.com/herb-cloves.html   Accessed on
January 30, 2016.
22. Herb Wisdom Website. Wormwood.
http://www.herbwisdom.com/herb-wormwood.html   Accessed
on January 30, 2016.
23. Superfood profiles website. Black Walnut
http://superfoodprofiles.com/black-walnut-benefits-health
Accessed on January 30, 2016.

Chapter 9: The Kidney Cleanse

1. National Kidney Foundation.
https://www.kidney.org/kidneydisease/howkidneyswrk
Accessed on January 26, 2016.
2. Wong, Cathy ND. Kidney Cleanse. Altmedicine website.
http://altmedicine.about.com/od/detoxcleansing/a/kidney_clea
nse.htm   Accessed on January 26, 2016.

Chapter 10: The Liver Cleanse

1. PubMed Health Website. Updated November 22, 2012.
http://www.ncbi.nlm.nih.gov/pubmedhealth/PMH0072577
Accessed on January 26, 2016.
2. Liver Cleanse. (n.d.). Retrieved from Dr. Clark's Legacy
Website
http://www.drhuldaclark.org/liver-cleanse

3. St. John, T. (2013). Defeat Cancer Now; A Nutritional Approach to Wellness for Cancer and Other Diseases. California: Alternative Health Solutions.
4. Coffee Enemas Reverses Cancer; By Waste Removal and Detoxifying. (n.d.). Treating Cancer Alternatively Website, Retrieved from http://www.treating-cancer-alternatively.com/Coffee-enemas.html
5. Wilson, L. Coffee Enemas: History & Benefits. (2012. April 21). Retrieved from Healing AIA Holistic Website http://www.healingaia.com/blog-resources/nutritional-balancing/five-elements-of-nutritional-balancing/detox-protocols/coffee-enemas

Chapter 11: Biofilms

1. "Frontline Hunting the Nightmare Bacteria" Documentary Frontline special 2013. Accessed from Netflix on December 19, 2015.
2. Arnold RS, Thom KA, Sharma S, Phillips M, Johnson JK, Morgan DJ. Emergence of *Klebsiella pneumoniae* Carbapenemase (KPC)-Producing Bacteria. *Southern medical journal*. 2011;104(1):40-45. doi:10.1097/SMJ.0b013e3181fd7d5a. http://www.ncbi.nlm.nih.gov/pmc/articles/PMC3075864
3. Steinberg, Doron, and Michael Friedman. 2000. "Development of Sustained-Release Devices for Modulation of Dental Plaque Biofilm and Treatment of Oral Infectious Diseases." *Drug Development Research* 50 (3-4): 555-565. doi:10.1002/1098-2299(200007/08)50:3/4<555: AID-DDR39>3.0.CO;2-P.
4. Dabbagh, Fatemeh, Manica Negahdaripour, Aydin Berenjian, Abdolazim Behfar, Fatemeh Mohammadi, Mozhdeh Zamani, Cambyz Irajie, and Younes Ghasemi. 2014. "Nattokinase: Production and Application." *Applied Microbiology and Biotechnology* 98 (22): 9199-9206. doi:10.1007/s00253-014-6135-3.
5. Versman, Heller, Beckman, "periodontal disease, heart disease and stroke." Periodontal Associates, no date given. http://www.periodontalhealth.com/procedures/periodontal-disease/periodontal-disease-heart-disease-and-stroke (accessed December 9, 2015).
6. Andy. "Using Serrapeptase to Control Bacterial Overgrowth Syndrome." Enzyme Therapies. No date given. http://enzymetherapies.com/20/serrapeptase/using-serrapeptase-to-control-bacterial-overgrowth-syndrome/# (accessed December 9, 2015).

7. Al-Bakri, A.G., G. Othman, and Y. Bustanji. 2009. "The assessment of the antibacterial and antifungal activities of aspirin, EDTA and aspirin-EDTA combination and their effectiveness as antibiofilm agents". *Journal of Applied Microbiology.* 107 (1): 280-286.

8. Banin E, Brady KM, Greenberg EP. Chelator-Induced Dispersal and Killing of *Pseudomonas aeruginosa* Cells in a Biofilm. *Applied and Environmental Microbiology.* 2006;72(3):2064-2069. doi:10.1128/AEM.72.3.2064-2069.2006.

9. Ammons MC, Copié V. Lactoferrin: A bioinspired, anti-biofilm therapeutic. *Biofouling.* 2013;29(4):443-455. doi:10.1080/08927014.2013.773317.

10. Jhajharia K, Parolia A, Shetty KV, Mehta LK. Biofilm in endodontics: A review. Journal of International Society of Preventive & Community Dentistry. 2015;5(1):1-12. doi:10.4103/2231-0762.151956.

11. Rajiv, S, Drilling A, Bassiouni A, James C, Vreugde S, Wormald PJ. International Forum of Allergy and Rhinology. Topical Colloidal Silver an anti-biofilm agent in a Staphylococcus aureus chronic rhinosinusitis sheep model. 2015 Apr;5(4):283-8. doi: 10.1002/alr.21459. Epub 2015 Jan 30.

12. Miao He, Minquan Du, Mingwen Fan, Zhuan Bian. In vitro activity of eugenol against Candida albicans biofilms. Mycopathologia, 2007, Volume 163, Number 3, Page 137.

13. Yadav MK[1], Chae SW[2], Im GJ[2], Chung JW[3], Song JJ[2]. PLoS One. 2015 Mar 17;10(3): e0119564. doi: 10.1371/journal.pone.0119564. eCollection 2015. Eugenol: a phyto-compound effective against methicillin-resistant and methicillin-sensitive Staphylococcus aureus clinical strain biofilms.

14. Dowd SE[1], Sun Y, Smith E, Kennedy JP, Jones CE, Wolcott R. Effects of biofilm treatments on the multi-species Lubbock chronic wound biofilm model. Journal of Wound Care. 2009 Dec;18(12):508, 510-12.

15. Yang, Liang, Yang Liu, Hong Wu, Zhijun Song, Niels Høiby, Søren Molin, and Michael Givskov. 2012. "Combating biofilms." *FEMS Immunology & Medical Microbiology* 65, no. 2: 146-157. *Environment Complete*, EBSCO*host* (accessed January 21, 2016).

16. érez-Giraldo, C., G. Cruz-Villalón, R. Sánchez-Silos, R. Martínez-Rubio, M.T. Blanco, and A.C. Gómez-García. 2003. "In vitro activity of allicin against Staphylococcus epidermidis and influence of sub inhibitory concentrations on biofilm

formation." *Journal of Applied Microbiology* 95, no. 4:
709. *Environment Complete,* EBSCO*host* (accessed January 21, 2016).
17. http://www.ncbi.nlm.nih.gov/pmc/articles/PMC3183659
Chandki, Rita, Priyank Banthia, and Ruchi Banthia. "Biofilms: A
Microbial Home." *Journal of Indian Society of Periodontology*
15.2 (2011): 111–114. *PMC.* Web. 29 Jan. 2016.
18. Schaller, James MD., Mountjoy, Kimberly. Combating
Biofilms; Why Your Antibiotics and Antifungals Fail.
International Infectious Disease Press, Florida. 2014.
19. Patel Thompson, Jini. Listen to your Gut. Caramal
Publishing. 2000-2012.
20. Georgetown University Medical Center. Oregano Oil May
Protect Against Drug-Resistant Bacteria, Georgetown
Researcher Finds. Science Daily. 2001 October 11. Accessed
on January 29, 2016.
21. Mark Force, William S. Sparks, Robert A. Ronzio. Inhibition
of enteric parasites by emulsified oil of oregano in vivo. Phyto
therapy Research. 200 May 11. vol.14 issue3 DOI:
10.1002/(SICI)1099-1573(200005)14:3<213: AID-
PTR583>3.0.CO;2-U.
22. Barrett, Mike. Health Benefits of Garlic-Anti-Cancer, Anti-
Infection, Detoxify and More. Written April 26, 2012.
http://naturalsociety.com/benefits-of-garlic   Accessed on
January 29, 2016.
23. Garlic and Cancer. http://www.cancer.gov/about-
cancer/causes-prevention/risk/diet/garlic-fact-sheet   Accessed
on January 29, 2016.
24. Tanalbit Product Page.
http://www.intensivenutrition.com/products/tanalbit-plant-
tannin-gi-support-product-120-capsules?variant=209996155
Accessed on January 29, 2016.
25. Moss, Ralph W. PhD. Herbs Against Cancer, History and
Controversy. Equinox Press, Inc. Brooklyn, New York. 1998.
26. Herb Wisdom. Com website. Herbal Benefits.
http://www.herbwisdom.com/herb-wormwood.html   Accessed
on January 29, 2016.
27. Mountain Rose Herbs website.
https://www.mountainroseherbs.com/products/oregon-grape-
root-extract/profile   Accessed on January 29, 2016.
28. Home Remedy Central Website. Oregon Grape Root
Extract. http://www.homeremedycentral.com/en/herbal-
remedies/extracts/oregon-grape-root-extract.html   Accessed
on January 29, 2016.

29. Applied Health Website.
http://appliedhealth.com/benefits-of-grapefruit-seed-extract
Accessed on January 29, 2016.
30. Herb Wisdom Website. Spirulina.
http://www.herbwisdom.com/herb-spirulina.html   Accessed on
January 30, 2016.
31. Herb Wisdom Website. Chlorella.
http://www.herbwisdom.com/herb-chlorella.html   Accessed on
January 30, 2016.
32. WebMD Website. NAC.
http://www.webmd.com/vitamins-
supplements/ingredientmono-1018-N-
ACETYL%20CYSTEINE.aspx?activeIngredientId=1018&activeIn
gredientName=N-ACETYL%20CYSTEINE   Accessed on January
31, 2016.
33. Tinnitus Website. NAC
http://tinnitushomepage.com/nac/nacaminoacid   Accessed on
January 31, 2016.
34. Fix Your Gut Website. NAG http://fixyourgut.com/three-
supplements-can-improve-integrity-digestive-system
Accessed on January 31, 2016.
35. Wong, Cathy ND. NAG. Altmedicine website.
http://altmedicine.about.com/od/glucosamine/a/N-Acetyl-
Glucosamine.htm Accessed on January 31, 2016.
36. Colostrum Website.
http://www.colostrummilk.com/colostrum-benefits   Accessed
on January 31, 2016.
37. Wyatt, Doug. Sovereign Laboratories Website.
http://www.sovereignlaboratories.com/info_THECOLOSTRUMMI
RACLE.html   Accessed on January 31, 2016.
38. Zehnder M. Root canal irrigants. J Endod. 2006; 32:389–
98.
39. Zamany A, Safavi K, Spångberg LS. The effect of
chlorhexidine as an endodontic disinfectant. Oral Surg Oral Med
Oral Pathol Oral Radiol Endod. 2003; 96:578–81.
40. Radcliffe CE, Potouridou L, Qureshi R, Habahbeh N,
Qualtrough A, Worthington H, et al. Antimicrobial activity of
varying concentrations of sodium hypochlorite on the
endodontic microorganisms Actinomyces israelii, A. naeslundii,
Candida albicans and Enterococcus faecalis. Int Endod J. 2004;
37:438–46.
41. Hwang BY, Roberts SK, Chadwick LR, Wu CD, Kinghorn
AD. Antimicrobial constituents from goldenseal (the Rhizomes
of Hydrastis canadensis) against selected oral pathogens.
Planta Med. 2003; 69:623–7.

42. Quan H, Cao YY, Xu Z, Zhao JX, Gao PH, Qin XF, et al. Potent *in vitro* synergism of fluconazole and berberine chloride against clinical isolates of Candida albicans resistant to fluconazole. Antimicrob Agents Chemother. 2006; 50:1096–9.
43. Imanshahidi M, Hosseinzadeh H. Pharmacological and therapeutic effects of Berberis vulgaris and its active constituent, berberine. Phytother Res. 2008; 22:999–1012.

Chapter 12: Juice Fasting
1. Manheim, J. (n.d.). Juicing vs. Blending. Retrieved from Healthy Green Drink Website.
 http://healthygreendrink.com/juicing-vs-blending/
2. Eat Goitrogens in Moderation and that includes Soy and Soya. (n.d.). Retrieved from
Stop the Thyroid Madness website from
http://www.stopthethyroidmadness.com/goitrogens
3. What are Goitrogens and what does it mean to the Hypothyroid. (n.d.). Retrieved from
 Hypothyroidism and Diet Information Website.
 http://www.hypothyroidismdietinfo.com/hypothyroidism-diet/hypothyroidism-diet-what-are-goitrogens.php
4. The Gerson Therapy. (2011. September 16). Retrieved from Gerson Clinic Website http://www.gerson.org
5. Walker. N.W. (1970). Fresh Vegetable and Fruit Juices. Arizona: Norwalk Press.
6. Fischer, W. (2000). How to Fight Cancer & Win. Maryland: Agora Health Books.
7. Harter Pierce, T. (2000). Outsmart Your Cancer; Alternative Non-Toxic Treatments That Work. Nevada: Thoughtworks Publishing.
8. St. John, T. (2013). Defeat Cancer Now; A Nutritional Approach to Wellness for Cancer and Other Diseases. California: Alternative Health Solutions.

Chapter 13: Water Fasting
1. Bragg, Patricia and Bragg, Paul. "The Miracle of Fasting". 53rd edition.

Chapter 14: Additional Detox Methods
1. St. John, Tamara. Website article "Miracle Pill that Should be in Every Household." http://tamarastjohn.com/miracle-pill-that-should-be-in-every-household   Accessed on January 31, 2016.

2. St. John, Tamara. Website article "Benefits of Oil Pulling." http://tamarastjohn.com/benefits-of-oil-pulling Accessed on October 24, 2016.
3. St. John, Tamara. Website article "How to Get Rid of a Toothache." http://tamarastjohn.com/get-rid-toothache Accessed on October 24, 2016.
4. St. John, T. (2013). Defeat Cancer Now; A Nutritional Approach to Wellness for Cancer and Other Diseases. California: Alternative Health Solutions.

Chapter 15: Detoxification Symptoms
1. Healthy Christian Living Website. Herxheimer Reaction. http://healthychristianliving.com/What%20Is%20The%20Herx heimer%20Reaction.htm   Accessed on January 30, 2016.
2. St. John, T. (2013). Defeat Cancer Now; A Nutritional Approach to Wellness for Cancer and Other Diseases. California: Alternative Health Solutions.

Chapter 18: Paleo Diet
1. Cordain, Loren Ph.D., The Paleo Diet Revised Edition 2011. John Wiley & Sons Inc.
2. Institute for Responsible Technology Website. http://nongmoshoppingguide.com/brands/invisible-gm-ingredients.html   Accessed January 29, 2016.

Chapter 19: GAPS Diet
1. Gaps Info Website. Gaps Introduction diet. http://www.gapsinfo.com/gaps-introduction-diet   Accessed January 26, 2016.
2. Campbell McBride, N. MD. GAPS; Gut and Psychology Syndrome.

Chapter 20: Ketogenic Diet
1. John's Hopkins Medical Center Website. Ketogenic Diet. http://www.hopkinsmedicine.org/neurology_neurosurgery/cent ers_clinics/epilepsy/pediatric_epilepsy/ketogenic_diet.html

Chapter 21: Vegan vs. Vegetarian
1. American Heart Association Website article on Vegetarian Diets.
http://www.heart.org/HEARTORG/HealthyLiving/HealthyEating/ Vegetarian-Diets_UCM_306032_Article.jsp#.Vq7YvrnSkfI Accessed on January 14, 2016.
2. Vegan.com website. http://www.vegan.com/what Accessed on January 14, 2016.

Chapter 22: Allergen Free Diets
1. Celiac website.
http://www.celiac.com/articles/182/1/Unsafe-Gluten-Free-Food-List-Unsafe-Ingredients/Page1.html   Accessed on January 29, 2016.
2. Institute for Responsible Technology Website. Genetically Modified Foods Ingredient List.
www.responsibletechnology.org   Accessed January 30, 2016.

Chapter 23: Low FODMAP Diet
1. Chris Kresser website. FODMAPs; Could Common Foods be Harming Your Digestive Health?
https://chriskresser.com/fodmaps-could-common-foods-be-harming-your-digestive-health/   Accessed March 12, 2017
2. Jacqueline S. Barrett, Peter R. Gibson. Fermentable oligosaccharides, disaccharides, monosaccharides and polyols (FODMAPs) and nonallergic food intolerance: FODMAPs or food chemicals? Therapeutic Advances in Gastroenterology. Vol 5, Issue 4, pp. 261 – 268. First published date: March-20-2012. Available from:
http://journals.sagepub.com/doi/abs/10.1177/1756283X11436241

Chapter 24: Extend Your Faith
1. Life Application Study Bible. New Living Translation.
        Illinois: Tyndale House Publishers, Inc.

Appendix A

My Favorites

The following is a list of my favorite products; the majority can be purchased on Amazon.com or Vitacost.com (unless noted otherwise) or ask for it in your local health food store.

Testing:
- Hair Mineral Analysis Testing & others: www.Unikeyhealth.com or call (800) 888-4353 M-F 7am to 5pm PST
- Adrenal profile, Stool Analysis, Food Intolerance www.labtestsplus.com
- pH strips
- ketogenic strips

Teas:
- Ginger Turmeric Herbal Tea (Trader Joe's)
- Moroccan Mint Tea Bags (Trader Joe's)
- Any herbal peppermint tea (check ingredients)
- Chocolate Mint Tea (Trader Joe's; seasonal)
- Teeccino herbal beverage (vitacost) in Hazelnut, Vanilla Nut, or gluten free varieties Dandelion Mocha Mint and Dandelion Caramel Nut (flavored coffee substitutes).
- Dandy Blend dandelion beverage (coffee substitute).

Foods:
- Mary's Gone Crackers Thins or Italian Style
- Silk Unsweetened Vanilla Almond Milk
- Silk Almond Milk Creamer (various flavors)
- Canyon Bakehouse Gluten Free, Allergen Free Bread
- Kerry Gold Butter
- Thai Kitchen Coconut Milk (full fat)
- Vitacost.com for many gluten free, non-GMO items low cost

Protein powders:
- Now Foods Pea Protein Powder; various flavors available

Supplements:
- Planetary Herbals Triphala Gold
- Planetary Herbals Stone Free
- Dr. Goodpet Food Grade Diatomaceous Earth
- Enema Kits: enema bags at local pharmacy
- North American Herb and Spice; Oregano Oil, Oregano Juice
- KyoGreen Powdered Drink Mix
- Navitas Naturals Maca Powder
- Nordic Naturals Arctic Cod Liver Oil capsules
- Atrantil (www.atrantil.com) also sells on Amazon.com
- Peppogest
- Humaworm (www.humaworm.com)
- Kirkland Parasite Cleansing Kit
- Symbiotics Candida Balance with Colostrum
- Trace Minerals Research; ConcenTrace Trace Mineral Drops (www.traceminerals.com)
- Grapefruit Seed Extract
- Seeking Health Histamine Block
- Nutricology DAO Histamine Digester
- Berberine (Vitacost brand)
- Quercetin/Bromelain (Vitacost brand)
- Doctor's Best Alpha Lipoic Acid 600 mg
- Standard Process Okra Pepsin E3
- Tanalbit
- Interphase Plus; Klaire Labs
- SF722; Thorne Research
- Serrapepidase; Doctors Best
- Nattokinase: Doctors Best
- Body Ecology liquid detox or candida detox (www.bodyecology.com)
- Natural Calm Magnesium Powder

Probiotics:
- Prescript Assist

- VSL #3
- Natren's

End Notes

It is my sincere hope that you found this book informative in your own healing process. To stay up to date with all my upcoming projects, book signings, speaking engagements, or to sign up for my newsletters, visit my website at www.Tamarastjohn.com or www.Tamarastjohn.org.

Other Published Books:

"Defeat Cancer Now" by Alternative Health Solutions publications. 2013. Available on my website, Amazon, Kindle, and Nook.

Author Biography

Tamara St. John is a full-time author, publisher and part-time professor living in the mountains of Southern California. She holds a Master's degree in Business Administration with a dual concentration in Accounting and Finance. It is this education which aided her in learning how to research meticulously in healing disease naturally.

In her spare time, she enjoys hiking, ice skating, and Disneyland.